JOURNALS

This journal belongs to:

_____

Strain

Grower _____ Date _____

Acquired _____ $ _____

THC % ____
CBD % ____

- [ ] Indica
- [ ] Sativa
- [ ] Hybrid

- [ ] Flower
- [ ] Edible
- [ ] Concentrate

Try again?
- [ ] Yes
- [ ] No

- [ ] Smoked
  - [ ] Rolled
  - [ ] Pipe
- [ ] Ate
- [ ] Dabbed
- [ ] Vaped

Symptoms Relieved

_____

_____

_____

_____

_____

Notes

_____

_____

_____

_____

_____

_____

Sweet

Fruity   Floral

Sour   Spicy

Earthy   Herbal

Woodsy

Effects	Strength				
Peaceful	○	○	○	○	○
Sleepy	○	○	○	○	○
Pain Relief	○	○	○	○	○
Hungry	○	○	○	○	○
Uplifted	○	○	○	○	○
Creative	○	○	○	○	○

Rating ☆ ☆ ☆ ☆ ☆

Strain _____

Grower _____   Date _____

Acquired _____ $ _____

THC % ___	☐ Indica	☐ Flower	Try again?
CBD % ___	☐ Sativa	☐ Edible	☐ Yes
	☐ Hybrid	☐ Concentrate	☐ No

☐ Smoked   ☐ Ate
  ☐ Rolled   ☐ Dabbed
  ☐ Pipe   ☐ Vaped

Symptoms Relieved

_____

_____

_____

_____

_____

Sweet

Fruity   Floral

Sour   Spicy

Earthy   Herbal

Woodsy

Notes

_____

_____

_____

_____

_____

_____

Effects	Strength				
Peaceful	○	○	○	○	○
Sleepy	○	○	○	○	○
Pain Relief	○	○	○	○	○
Hungry	○	○	○	○	○
Uplifted	○	○	○	○	○
Creative	○	○	○	○	○

Rating ☆ ☆ ☆ ☆ ☆

Strain _____

Grower _____ Date _____

Acquired _____ $ _____

| THC % ____ CBD % ____ | ☐ Indica ☐ Sativa ☐ Hybrid | ☐ Flower ☐ Edible ☐ Concentrate | Try again? ☐ Yes ☐ No |

☐ Smoked   ☐ Ate
   ☐ Rolled   ☐ Dabbed
   ☐ Pipe   ☐ Vaped

Symptoms Relieved

_____

_____

_____

_____

Notes

_____

_____

_____

_____

_____

_____

Sweet
Fruity   Floral
Sour   Spicy
Earthy   Herbal
Woodsy

Effects	Strength
Peaceful	○ ○ ○ ○ ○
Sleepy	○ ○ ○ ○ ○
Pain Relief	○ ○ ○ ○ ○
Hungry	○ ○ ○ ○ ○
Uplifted	○ ○ ○ ○ ○
Creative	○ ○ ○ ○ ○

Rating ☆ ☆ ☆ ☆ ☆

Strain _____

Grower _____ Date _____

Acquired _____ $ _____

THC % ____	☐ Indica	☐ Flower	Try again?
CBD % ____	☐ Sativa	☐ Edible	☐ Yes
	☐ Hybrid	☐ Concentrate	☐ No

☐ Smoked   ☐ Ate
  ☐ Rolled   ☐ Dabbed
  ☐ Pipe   ☐ Vaped

Sweet

Fruity   Floral

Sour   Spicy

Earthy   Herbal

Woodsy

Symptoms Relieved

_____

_____

_____

_____

_____

Notes

_____

_____

_____

_____

_____

_____

Effects	Strength				
Peaceful	○	○	○	○	○
Sleepy	○	○	○	○	○
Pain Relief	○	○	○	○	○
Hungry	○	○	○	○	○
Uplifted	○	○	○	○	○
Creative	○	○	○	○	○

Rating ☆ ☆ ☆ ☆ ☆

Strain

Grower _____ Date _____

Acquired _____ $ _____

THC % ____
CBD % ____

- [ ] Indica
- [ ] Sativa
- [ ] Hybrid

- [ ] Flower
- [ ] Edible
- [ ] Concentrate

Try again?
- [ ] Yes
- [ ] No

- [ ] Smoked
  - [ ] Rolled
  - [ ] Pipe
- [ ] Ate
- [ ] Dabbed
- [ ] Vaped

Symptoms Relieved

_____

_____

_____

_____

_____

Sweet

Fruity   Floral

Sour   Spicy

Earthy   Herbal

Woodsy

Notes

_____

_____

_____

_____

_____

_____

Effects	Strength				
Peaceful	○	○	○	○	○
Sleepy	○	○	○	○	○
Pain Relief	○	○	○	○	○
Hungry	○	○	○	○	○
Uplifted	○	○	○	○	○
Creative	○	○	○	○	○

Rating ☆ ☆ ☆ ☆ ☆

Strain _____

Grower _____   Date _____

Acquired _____ $ _____

THC % ____	☐ Indica	☐ Flower	Try again?
CBD % ____	☐ Sativa	☐ Edible	☐ Yes
	☐ Hybrid	☐ Concentrate	☐ No

☐ Smoked   ☐ Ate
  ☐ Rolled   ☐ Dabbed
  ☐ Pipe   ☐ Vaped

Symptoms Relieved

_____

_____

_____

_____

_____

Sweet

Fruity   Floral

Sour   Spicy

Earthy   Herbal

Woodsy

Notes

_____

_____

_____

_____

_____

Effects	Strength
Peaceful	○ ○ ○ ○ ○
Sleepy	○ ○ ○ ○ ○
Pain Relief	○ ○ ○ ○ ○
Hungry	○ ○ ○ ○ ○
Uplifted	○ ○ ○ ○ ○
Creative	○ ○ ○ ○ ○

Rating ☆ ☆ ☆ ☆ ☆

Strain

Grower _____ Date _____

Acquired _____ $ _____

THC % ___	☐ Indica	☐ Flower	Try again?
CBD % ___	☐ Sativa	☐ Edible	☐ Yes
	☐ Hybrid	☐ Concentrate	☐ No

☐ Smoked   ☐ Ate
   ☐ Rolled   ☐ Dabbed
   ☐ Pipe   ☐ Vaped

Symptoms Relieved

_____

_____

_____

_____

_____

Sweet
Fruity   Floral
Sour   Spicy
Earthy   Herbal
Woodsy

Notes

_____

_____

_____

_____

_____

_____

Effects	Strength
Peaceful	○ ○ ○ ○ ○
Sleepy	○ ○ ○ ○ ○
Pain Relief	○ ○ ○ ○ ○
Hungry	○ ○ ○ ○ ○
Uplifted	○ ○ ○ ○ ○
Creative	○ ○ ○ ○ ○

Rating ☆ ☆ ☆ ☆ ☆

Strain _____

Grower _____   Date _____

Acquired _____ $ _____

THC % ___	☐ Indica	☐ Flower	Try again?
CBD % ___	☐ Sativa	☐ Edible	☐ Yes
	☐ Hybrid	☐ Concentrate	☐ No

☐ Smoked   ☐ Ate
  ☐ Rolled   ☐ Dabbed
  ☐ Pipe   ☐ Vaped

Sweet

Fruity   Floral

Sour   Spicy

Earthy   Herbal

Woodsy

Symptoms Relieved

_____

_____

_____

_____

_____

Effects	Strength
Peaceful	○ ○ ○ ○ ○
Sleepy	○ ○ ○ ○ ○
Pain Relief	○ ○ ○ ○ ○
Hungry	○ ○ ○ ○ ○
Uplifted	○ ○ ○ ○ ○
Creative	○ ○ ○ ○ ○

Notes

_____

_____

_____

_____

_____

_____

Rating ☆ ☆ ☆ ☆ ☆

Strain _____

Grower _____   Date _____

Acquired _____ $ _____

THC % ___	☐ Indica	☐ Flower	Try again?
CBD % ___	☐ Sativa	☐ Edible	☐ Yes
	☐ Hybrid	☐ Concentrate	☐ No

☐ Smoked   ☐ Ate
  ☐ Rolled   ☐ Dabbed
  ☐ Pipe   ☐ Vaped

Symptoms Relieved

_____

_____

_____

_____

_____

Notes

_____

_____

_____

_____

_____

_____

Sweet

Fruity   Floral

Sour   Spicy

Earthy   Herbal

Woodsy

Effects	Strength				
Peaceful	○	○	○	○	○
Sleepy	○	○	○	○	○
Pain Relief	○	○	○	○	○
Hungry	○	○	○	○	○
Uplifted	○	○	○	○	○
Creative	○	○	○	○	○

Rating ☆ ☆ ☆ ☆ ☆

Strain _____

Grower _____   Date _____

Acquired _____ $ _____

THC % ____	☐ Indica	☐ Flower	Try again?
CBD % ____	☐ Sativa	☐ Edible	☐ Yes
	☐ Hybrid	☐ Concentrate	☐ No

☐ Smoked   ☐ Ate
  ☐ Rolled   ☐ Dabbed
  ☐ Pipe   ☐ Vaped

Sweet

Fruity   Floral

Sour   Spicy

Earthy   Herbal

Woodsy

Symptoms Relieved

_____

_____

_____

_____

_____

Notes

_____

_____

_____

_____

_____

_____

Effects	Strength
Peaceful	○ ○ ○ ○ ○
Sleepy	○ ○ ○ ○ ○
Pain Relief	○ ○ ○ ○ ○
Hungry	○ ○ ○ ○ ○
Uplifted	○ ○ ○ ○ ○
Creative	○ ○ ○ ○ ○

Rating ☆ ☆ ☆ ☆ ☆

Strain _____

Grower _____   Date _____

Acquired _____ $ _____

THC % ____	☐ Indica	☐ Flower	Try again?
CBD % ____	☐ Sativa	☐ Edible	☐ Yes
	☐ Hybrid	☐ Concentrate	☐ No

☐ Smoked   ☐ Ate
  ☐ Rolled   ☐ Dabbed
  ☐ Pipe   ☐ Vaped

Symptoms Relieved

_____

_____

_____

_____

_____

Notes

_____

_____

_____

_____

_____

_____

Sweet

Fruity   Floral

Sour   Spicy

Earthy   Herbal

Woodsy

Effects	Strength
Peaceful	○ ○ ○ ○ ○
Sleepy	○ ○ ○ ○ ○
Pain Relief	○ ○ ○ ○ ○
Hungry	○ ○ ○ ○ ○
Uplifted	○ ○ ○ ○ ○
Creative	○ ○ ○ ○ ○

Rating ☆ ☆ ☆ ☆ ☆

Strain _____

Grower _____ Date _____

Acquired _____ $ _____

THC % ___	☐ Indica	☐ Flower	**Try again?**
CBD % ___	☐ Sativa	☐ Edible	☐ Yes
	☐ Hybrid	☐ Concentrate	☐ No

☐ Smoked   ☐ Ate
  ☐ Rolled   ☐ Dabbed
  ☐ Pipe   ☐ Vaped

Symptoms Relieved

_____

_____

_____

_____

_____

Notes

_____

_____

_____

_____

_____

Sweet

Fruity   Floral

Sour   Spicy

Earthy   Herbal

Woodsy

Effects	**Strength**
Peaceful	○ ○ ○ ○ ○
Sleepy	○ ○ ○ ○ ○
Pain Relief	○ ○ ○ ○ ○
Hungry	○ ○ ○ ○ ○
Uplifted	○ ○ ○ ○ ○
Creative	○ ○ ○ ○ ○

Rating ☆ ☆ ☆ ☆ ☆

Strain

Grower _____ Date _____

Acquired _____ $ _____

THC % ____
CBD % ____

- [ ] Indica
- [ ] Sativa
- [ ] Hybrid

- [ ] Flower
- [ ] Edible
- [ ] Concentrate

Try again?
- [ ] Yes
- [ ] No

- [ ] Smoked
  - [ ] Rolled
  - [ ] Pipe
- [ ] Ate
- [ ] Dabbed
- [ ] Vaped

Symptoms Relieved

_____

_____

_____

_____

_____

Notes

_____

_____

_____

_____

_____

_____

_____

Sweet

Fruity · Floral

Sour · Spicy

Earthy · Herbal

Woodsy

Effects	Strength
Peaceful	○ ○ ○ ○ ○
Sleepy	○ ○ ○ ○ ○
Pain Relief	○ ○ ○ ○ ○
Hungry	○ ○ ○ ○ ○
Uplifted	○ ○ ○ ○ ○
Creative	○ ○ ○ ○ ○

Rating ☆ ☆ ☆ ☆ ☆

Strain _____

Grower _____ Date _____

Acquired _____ $ _____

THC % ___	☐ Indica	☐ Flower	Try again?
CBD % ___	☐ Sativa	☐ Edible	☐ Yes
	☐ Hybrid	☐ Concentrate	☐ No

☐ Smoked   ☐ Ate
　☐ Rolled   ☐ Dabbed
　☐ Pipe   ☐ Vaped

Symptoms Relieved

_____

_____

_____

_____

_____

Notes

_____

_____

_____

_____

_____

_____

Sweet

Fruity   Floral

Sour   Spicy

Earthy   Herbal

Woodsy

Effects	Strength
Peaceful	○ ○ ○ ○ ○
Sleepy	○ ○ ○ ○ ○
Pain Relief	○ ○ ○ ○ ○
Hungry	○ ○ ○ ○ ○
Uplifted	○ ○ ○ ○ ○
Creative	○ ○ ○ ○ ○

Rating ☆ ☆ ☆ ☆ ☆

Strain _____

Grower _____ Date _____

Acquired _____ $ _____

| THC % ___
CBD % ___ | ☐ Indica
☐ Sativa
☐ Hybrid | ☐ Flower
☐ Edible
☐ Concentrate | Try again?
☐ Yes
☐ No |

| ☐ Smoked   ☐ Ate |
| ☐ Rolled   ☐ Dabbed |
| ☐ Pipe   ☐ Vaped |

Sweet

Fruity   Floral

Sour   Spicy

Earthy   Herbal

Woodsy

Symptoms Relieved

_____

_____

_____

_____

_____

Effects	Strength
Peaceful	○ ○ ○ ○ ○
Sleepy	○ ○ ○ ○ ○
Pain Relief	○ ○ ○ ○ ○
Hungry	○ ○ ○ ○ ○
Uplifted	○ ○ ○ ○ ○
Creative	○ ○ ○ ○ ○

Notes

_____

_____

_____

_____

_____

_____

Rating ☆ ☆ ☆ ☆ ☆

Strain _____

Grower _____   Date _____

Acquired _____ $ _____

THC % ___	☐ Indica
CBD % ___	☐ Sativa
	☐ Hybrid

☐ Flower
☐ Edible
☐ Concentrate

Try again?
☐ Yes
☐ No

☐ Smoked   ☐ Ate
   ☐ Rolled   ☐ Dabbed
   ☐ Pipe   ☐ Vaped

Symptoms Relieved

_____

_____

_____

_____

_____

Notes

_____

_____

_____

_____

_____

_____

_____

Sweet

Fruity

Floral

Sour

Spicy

Earthy

Herbal

Woodsy

Effects	Strength
Peaceful	○ ○ ○ ○ ○
Sleepy	○ ○ ○ ○ ○
Pain Relief	○ ○ ○ ○ ○
Hungry	○ ○ ○ ○ ○
Uplifted	○ ○ ○ ○ ○
Creative	○ ○ ○ ○ ○

Rating ☆ ☆ ☆ ☆ ☆

Strain _____

Grower _____   Date _____

Acquired _____ $ _____

THC % ____	☐ Indica	☐ Flower	Try again?
CBD % ____	☐ Sativa	☐ Edible	☐ Yes
	☐ Hybrid	☐ Concentrate	☐ No

☐ Smoked   ☐ Ate
  ☐ Rolled   ☐ Dabbed
  ☐ Pipe   ☐ Vaped

Symptoms Relieved

_____

_____

_____

_____

Notes

_____

_____

_____

_____

_____

Sweet
Fruity   Floral
Sour   Spicy
Earthy   Herbal
Woodsy

Effects	Strength
Peaceful	○ ○ ○ ○ ○
Sleepy	○ ○ ○ ○ ○
Pain Relief	○ ○ ○ ○ ○
Hungry	○ ○ ○ ○ ○
Uplifted	○ ○ ○ ○ ○
Creative	○ ○ ○ ○ ○

Rating ☆ ☆ ☆ ☆ ☆

Strain _____

Grower _____ Date _____

Acquired _____ $ _____

THC % ___	☐ Indica	☐ Flower	Try again?
CBD % ___	☐ Sativa	☐ Edible	☐ Yes
	☐ Hybrid	☐ Concentrate	☐ No

☐ Smoked   ☐ Ate
  ☐ Rolled   ☐ Dabbed
  ☐ Pipe   ☐ Vaped

Sweet

Fruity   Floral

Sour   Spicy

Symptoms Relieved

_____

_____   Earthy   Herbal

_____

_____   Woodsy

_____

Effects	Strength				
Peaceful	○	○	○	○	○
Sleepy	○	○	○	○	○
Pain Relief	○	○	○	○	○
Hungry	○	○	○	○	○
Uplifted	○	○	○	○	○
Creative	○	○	○	○	○

Notes

_____

_____

_____

_____

_____   **Rating** ☆ ☆ ☆ ☆ ☆

_____

Strain

Grower _____ Date _____

Acquired _____ $ _____

THC % _____
CBD % _____

- [ ] Indica
- [ ] Sativa
- [ ] Hybrid

- [ ] Flower
- [ ] Edible
- [ ] Concentrate

Try again?
- [ ] Yes
- [ ] No

- [ ] Smoked
  - [ ] Rolled
  - [ ] Pipe
- [ ] Ate
- [ ] Dabbed
- [ ] Vaped

Symptoms Relieved

_____

_____

_____

_____

_____

Sweet

Fruity   Floral

Sour   Spicy

Earthy   Herbal

Woodsy

Notes

_____

_____

_____

_____

_____

_____

_____

Effects	Strength				
Peaceful	○	○	○	○	○
Sleepy	○	○	○	○	○
Pain Relief	○	○	○	○	○
Hungry	○	○	○	○	○
Uplifted	○	○	○	○	○
Creative	○	○	○	○	○

Rating ☆ ☆ ☆ ☆ ☆

Strain _____

Grower _____ Date _____

Acquired _____ $ _____

THC % ____
CBD % ____

☐ Indica
☐ Sativa
☐ Hybrid

☐ Flower
☐ Edible
☐ Concentrate

Try again?
☐ Yes
☐ No

☐ Smoked
　☐ Rolled
　☐ Pipe

☐ Ate
☐ Dabbed
☐ Vaped

Symptoms Relieved

_____

_____

_____

_____

_____

Notes

_____

_____

_____

_____

_____

_____

Sweet

Fruity　　　　　　Floral

Sour　　　　　　Spicy

Earthy　　　　　　Herbal

Woodsy

Effects	Strength				
Peaceful	○	○	○	○	○
Sleepy	○	○	○	○	○
Pain Relief	○	○	○	○	○
Hungry	○	○	○	○	○
Uplifted	○	○	○	○	○
Creative	○	○	○	○	○

Rating ☆ ☆ ☆ ☆ ☆

Strain _____

Grower _____   Date _____

Acquired _____ $ _____

THC % ____
CBD % ____

- [ ] Indica
- [ ] Sativa
- [ ] Hybrid

- [ ] Flower
- [ ] Edible
- [ ] Concentrate

Try again?
- [ ] Yes
- [ ] No

- [ ] Smoked
  - [ ] Rolled
  - [ ] Pipe
- [ ] Ate
- [ ] Dabbed
- [ ] Vaped

Symptoms Relieved

_____

_____

_____

_____

_____

Notes

_____

_____

_____

_____

_____

_____

Sweet
Fruity   Floral
Sour   Spicy
Earthy   Herbal
Woodsy

Effects	Strength				
Peaceful	○	○	○	○	○
Sleepy	○	○	○	○	○
Pain Relief	○	○	○	○	○
Hungry	○	○	○	○	○
Uplifted	○	○	○	○	○
Creative	○	○	○	○	○

Rating ☆ ☆ ☆ ☆ ☆

Strain _____

Grower _____ Date _____

Acquired _____ $ _____

THC % ____	☐ Indica	☐ Flower	**Try again?**
CBD % ____	☐ Sativa	☐ Edible	☐ Yes
	☐ Hybrid	☐ Concentrate	☐ No

☐ Smoked   ☐ Ate
  ☐ Rolled   ☐ Dabbed
  ☐ Pipe   ☐ Vaped

Symptoms Relieved

_____

_____

_____

_____

_____

Notes

_____

_____

_____

_____

_____

_____

Sweet

Fruity   Floral

Sour   Spicy

Earthy   Herbal

Woodsy

Effects	Strength				
Peaceful	○	○	○	○	○
Sleepy	○	○	○	○	○
Pain Relief	○	○	○	○	○
Hungry	○	○	○	○	○
Uplifted	○	○	○	○	○
Creative	○	○	○	○	○

Rating ☆ ☆ ☆ ☆ ☆

Strain

Grower _____ Date _____

Acquired _____ $ _____

THC % ____
CBD % ____

- [ ] Indica
- [ ] Sativa
- [ ] Hybrid

- [ ] Flower
- [ ] Edible
- [ ] Concentrate

Try again?
- [ ] Yes
- [ ] No

- [ ] Smoked
  - [ ] Rolled
  - [ ] Pipe
- [ ] Ate
- [ ] Dabbed
- [ ] Vaped

Symptoms Relieved

_____

_____

_____

_____

Notes

_____

_____

_____

_____

_____

_____

Sweet

Fruity

Floral

Sour

Spicy

Earthy

Herbal

Woodsy

Effects	Strength				
Peaceful	○	○	○	○	○
Sleepy	○	○	○	○	○
Pain Relief	○	○	○	○	○
Hungry	○	○	○	○	○
Uplifted	○	○	○	○	○
Creative	○	○	○	○	○

Rating ☆ ☆ ☆ ☆ ☆

Strain _____

Grower _____ Date _____

Acquired _____ $ _____

THC % ____	☐ Indica	☐ Flower	Try again?
CBD % ____	☐ Sativa	☐ Edible	☐ Yes
	☐ Hybrid	☐ Concentrate	☐ No

☐ Smoked   ☐ Ate
  ☐ Rolled   ☐ Dabbed
  ☐ Pipe   ☐ Vaped

Symptoms Relieved

_____

_____

_____

_____

Notes

_____

_____

_____

_____

_____

Sweet
Fruity   Floral
Sour   Spicy
Earthy   Herbal
Woodsy

Effects	Strength
Peaceful	○ ○ ○ ○ ○
Sleepy	○ ○ ○ ○ ○
Pain Relief	○ ○ ○ ○ ○
Hungry	○ ○ ○ ○ ○
Uplifted	○ ○ ○ ○ ○
Creative	○ ○ ○ ○ ○

Rating ☆ ☆ ☆ ☆ ☆

Strain

Grower _____ Date _____

Acquired _____ $ _____

THC % _____
CBD % _____

- [ ] Indica
- [ ] Sativa
- [ ] Hybrid

- [ ] Flower
- [ ] Edible
- [ ] Concentrate

Try again?
- [ ] Yes
- [ ] No

- [ ] Smoked
  - [ ] Rolled
  - [ ] Pipe
- [ ] Ate
- [ ] Dabbed
- [ ] Vaped

Symptoms Relieved

_____

_____

_____

_____

_____

Sweet

Fruity

Floral

Sour

Spicy

Earthy

Herbal

Woodsy

Notes

_____

_____

_____

_____

_____

_____

Effects	Strength				
Peaceful	○	○	○	○	○
Sleepy	○	○	○	○	○
Pain Relief	○	○	○	○	○
Hungry	○	○	○	○	○
Uplifted	○	○	○	○	○
Creative	○	○	○	○	○

Rating ☆ ☆ ☆ ☆ ☆

Strain _____

Grower _____   Date _____

Acquired _____ $ _____

THC % ___	☐ Indica
CBD % ___	☐ Sativa
	☐ Hybrid

☐ Flower
☐ Edible
☐ Concentrate

Try again?
☐ Yes
☐ No

☐ Smoked   ☐ Ate
　☐ Rolled   ☐ Dabbed
　☐ Pipe   ☐ Vaped

Sweet

Fruity　　　　　Floral

Sour　　　　　Spicy

Earthy　　　　Herbal

Woodsy

Symptoms Relieved

_____

_____

_____

_____

_____

Effects	Strength
Peaceful	◯ ◯ ◯ ◯ ◯
Sleepy	◯ ◯ ◯ ◯ ◯
Pain Relief	◯ ◯ ◯ ◯ ◯
Hungry	◯ ◯ ◯ ◯ ◯
Uplifted	◯ ◯ ◯ ◯ ◯
Creative	◯ ◯ ◯ ◯ ◯

Notes

_____

_____

_____

_____

_____

Rating ☆ ☆ ☆ ☆ ☆

Strain _____

Grower _____   Date _____

Acquired _____ $ _____

THC % ___ CBD % ___	☐ Indica ☐ Sativa ☐ Hybrid	☐ Flower ☐ Edible ☐ Concentrate	Try again? ☐ Yes ☐ No

☐ Smoked   ☐ Ate
☐ Rolled   ☐ Dabbed
☐ Pipe   ☐ Vaped

Symptoms Relieved

_____
_____
_____
_____
_____

Notes

_____
_____
_____
_____
_____
_____

Sweet

Fruity   Floral

Sour   Spicy

Earthy   Herbal

Woodsy

Effects	Strength
Peaceful	○ ○ ○ ○ ○
Sleepy	○ ○ ○ ○ ○
Pain Relief	○ ○ ○ ○ ○
Hungry	○ ○ ○ ○ ○
Uplifted	○ ○ ○ ○ ○
Creative	○ ○ ○ ○ ○

Rating ☆ ☆ ☆ ☆ ☆

Strain _____

Grower _____ Date _____

Acquired _____ $ _____

THC % ____	☐ Indica	☐ Flower	Try again?
	☐ Sativa	☐ Edible	☐ Yes
CBD % ____	☐ Hybrid	☐ Concentrate	☐ No

☐ Smoked   ☐ Ate
☐ Rolled   ☐ Dabbed
☐ Pipe   ☐ Vaped

Symptoms Relieved

_____

_____

_____

_____

_____

Sweet

Fruity   Floral

Sour   Spicy

Earthy   Herbal

Woodsy

Notes

_____

_____

_____

_____

_____

_____

Effects	Strength
Peaceful	○ ○ ○ ○ ○
Sleepy	○ ○ ○ ○ ○
Pain Relief	○ ○ ○ ○ ○
Hungry	○ ○ ○ ○ ○
Uplifted	○ ○ ○ ○ ○
Creative	○ ○ ○ ○ ○

Rating ☆ ☆ ☆ ☆ ☆

Strain _____

Grower _____   Date _____

Acquired _____ $ _____

THC % ____ CBD % ____	☐ Indica ☐ Sativa ☐ Hybrid	☐ Flower ☐ Edible ☐ Concentrate	**Try again?** ☐ Yes ☐ No	

☐ Smoked   ☐ Ate
   ☐ Rolled   ☐ Dabbed
   ☐ Pipe   ☐ Vaped

Symptoms Relieved

_____

_____

_____

_____

_____

Notes

_____

_____

_____

_____

_____

_____

Sweet
Fruity   Floral
Sour   Spicy
Earthy   Herbal
Woodsy

Effects	Strength				
Peaceful	○	○	○	○	○
Sleepy	○	○	○	○	○
Pain Relief	○	○	○	○	○
Hungry	○	○	○	○	○
Uplifted	○	○	○	○	○
Creative	○	○	○	○	○

Rating ☆ ☆ ☆ ☆ ☆

Strain _____

Grower _____ Date _____

Acquired _____ $ _____

THC % ____
CBD % ____

- [ ] Indica
- [ ] Sativa
- [ ] Hybrid

- [ ] Flower
- [ ] Edible
- [ ] Concentrate

Try again?
- [ ] Yes
- [ ] No

- [ ] Smoked
  - [ ] Rolled
  - [ ] Pipe
- [ ] Ate
- [ ] Dabbed
- [ ] Vaped

Symptoms Relieved

_____

_____

_____

_____

Notes

_____

_____

_____

_____

_____

Sweet
Fruity
Floral
Sour
Spicy
Earthy
Herbal
Woodsy

Effects	Strength				
Peaceful	○	○	○	○	○
Sleepy	○	○	○	○	○
Pain Relief	○	○	○	○	○
Hungry	○	○	○	○	○
Uplifted	○	○	○	○	○
Creative	○	○	○	○	○

Rating ☆ ☆ ☆ ☆ ☆

Strain _____

Grower _____ Date _____

Acquired _____ $ _____

| THC % ____ CBD % ____ | ☐ Indica ☐ Sativa ☐ Hybrid | ☐ Flower ☐ Edible ☐ Concentrate | Try again? ☐ Yes ☐ No |

☐ Smoked
  ☐ Rolled
  ☐ Pipe
☐ Ate
☐ Dabbed
☐ Vaped

Symptoms Relieved

_____

_____

_____

_____

_____

Notes

_____

_____

_____

_____

_____

_____

Sweet
Fruity   Floral
Sour   Spicy
Earthy   Herbal
Woodsy

Effects	Strength
Peaceful	○ ○ ○ ○ ○
Sleepy	○ ○ ○ ○ ○
Pain Relief	○ ○ ○ ○ ○
Hungry	○ ○ ○ ○ ○
Uplifted	○ ○ ○ ○ ○
Creative	○ ○ ○ ○ ○

Rating ☆ ☆ ☆ ☆ ☆

Strain _____

Grower _____ Date _____

Acquired _____ $ _____

| THC % ____
CBD % ____ | ☐ Indica
☐ Sativa
☐ Hybrid | ☐ Flower
☐ Edible
☐ Concentrate | **Try again?**
☐ Yes
☐ No |

☐ Smoked   ☐ Ate
  ☐ Rolled   ☐ Dabbed
  ☐ Pipe   ☐ Vaped

Symptoms Relieved

_____

_____

_____

_____

_____

Notes

_____

_____

_____

_____

_____

_____

Sweet

Fruity   Floral

Sour   Spicy

Earthy   Herbal

Woodsy

Effects	Strength				
Peaceful	○	○	○	○	○
Sleepy	○	○	○	○	○
Pain Relief	○	○	○	○	○
Hungry	○	○	○	○	○
Uplifted	○	○	○	○	○
Creative	○	○	○	○	○

Rating ☆ ☆ ☆ ☆ ☆

Strain _____

Grower _____ Date _____

Acquired _____ $ _____

THC % ___	☐ Indica	☐ Flower	Try again?
CBD % ___	☐ Sativa	☐ Edible	☐ Yes
	☐ Hybrid	☐ Concentrate	☐ No

☐ Smoked   ☐ Ate
  ☐ Rolled   ☐ Dabbed
  ☐ Pipe   ☐ Vaped

Symptoms Relieved

_____

_____

_____

_____

Sweet

Fruity   Floral

Sour   Spicy

Earthy   Herbal

Woodsy

Notes

_____

_____

_____

_____

_____

_____

Effects	Strength				
Peaceful	○	○	○	○	○
Sleepy	○	○	○	○	○
Pain Relief	○	○	○	○	○
Hungry	○	○	○	○	○
Uplifted	○	○	○	○	○
Creative	○	○	○	○	○

Rating ☆ ☆ ☆ ☆ ☆

Strain

Grower _____ Date _____

Acquired _____ $ _____

THC % ___
CBD % ___

- [ ] Indica
- [ ] Sativa
- [ ] Hybrid

- [ ] Flower
- [ ] Edible
- [ ] Concentrate

Try again?
- [ ] Yes
- [ ] No

- [ ] Smoked
  - [ ] Rolled
  - [ ] Pipe
- [ ] Ate
- [ ] Dabbed
- [ ] Vaped

Symptoms Relieved

_____

_____

_____

_____

_____

Notes

_____

_____

_____

_____

_____

_____

Sweet

Fruity   Floral

Sour   Spicy

Earthy   Herbal

Woodsy

Effects	Strength				
Peaceful	○	○	○	○	○
Sleepy	○	○	○	○	○
Pain Relief	○	○	○	○	○
Hungry	○	○	○	○	○
Uplifted	○	○	○	○	○
Creative	○	○	○	○	○

Rating ☆ ☆ ☆ ☆ ☆

Strain _____

Grower _____ Date _____

Acquired _____ $ _____

THC % ____	☐ Indica	☐ Flower	Try again?
CBD % ____	☐ Sativa	☐ Edible	☐ Yes
	☐ Hybrid	☐ Concentrate	☐ No

☐ Smoked ☐ Ate
  ☐ Rolled ☐ Dabbed
  ☐ Pipe ☐ Vaped

Symptoms Relieved

_____

_____

_____

_____

_____

Notes

_____

_____

_____

_____

_____

_____

_____

Sweet
Fruity   Floral
Sour   Spicy
Earthy   Herbal
Woodsy

Effects	Strength
Peaceful	○ ○ ○ ○ ○
Sleepy	○ ○ ○ ○ ○
Pain Relief	○ ○ ○ ○ ○
Hungry	○ ○ ○ ○ ○
Uplifted	○ ○ ○ ○ ○
Creative	○ ○ ○ ○ ○

Rating ☆ ☆ ☆ ☆ ☆

Strain _____

Grower _____ Date _____

Acquired _____ $ _____

THC % ___	☐ Indica	☐ Flower	Try again?
CBD % ___	☐ Sativa	☐ Edible	☐ Yes
	☐ Hybrid	☐ Concentrate	☐ No

☐ Smoked   ☐ Ate
  ☐ Rolled   ☐ Dabbed
  ☐ Pipe   ☐ Vaped

Symptoms Relieved

_____
_____
_____
_____

Sweet
Fruity   Floral
Sour   Spicy
Earthy   Herbal
Woodsy

Notes

_____
_____
_____
_____
_____

Effects	Strength				
Peaceful	○	○	○	○	○
Sleepy	○	○	○	○	○
Pain Relief	○	○	○	○	○
Hungry	○	○	○	○	○
Uplifted	○	○	○	○	○
Creative	○	○	○	○	○

Rating ☆ ☆ ☆ ☆ ☆

Strain _____

Grower _____ Date _____

Acquired _____ $ _____

THC % ____

CBD % ____

- [ ] Indica
- [ ] Sativa
- [ ] Hybrid

- [ ] Flower
- [ ] Edible
- [ ] Concentrate

Try again?
- [ ] Yes
- [ ] No

- [ ] Smoked
  - [ ] Rolled
  - [ ] Pipe
- [ ] Ate
- [ ] Dabbed
- [ ] Vaped

Symptoms Relieved

_____

_____

_____

_____

_____

Notes

_____

_____

_____

_____

_____

_____

Sweet

Fruity

Floral

Sour

Spicy

Earthy

Herbal

Woodsy

Effects	Strength				
Peaceful	○	○	○	○	○
Sleepy	○	○	○	○	○
Pain Relief	○	○	○	○	○
Hungry	○	○	○	○	○
Uplifted	○	○	○	○	○
Creative	○	○	○	○	○

Rating ☆ ☆ ☆ ☆ ☆

Strain _____

Grower _____ Date _____

Acquired _____ $ _____

THC % ____
CBD % ____

- [ ] Indica
- [ ] Sativa
- [ ] Hybrid

- [ ] Flower
- [ ] Edible
- [ ] Concentrate

Try again?
- [ ] Yes
- [ ] No

- [ ] Smoked
  - [ ] Rolled
  - [ ] Pipe
- [ ] Ate
- [ ] Dabbed
- [ ] Vaped

Symptoms Relieved

_____

_____

_____

_____

_____

Notes

_____

_____

_____

_____

_____

_____

Sweet

Fruity   Floral

Sour   Spicy

Earthy   Herbal

Woodsy

Effects	Strength				
Peaceful	○	○	○	○	○
Sleepy	○	○	○	○	○
Pain Relief	○	○	○	○	○
Hungry	○	○	○	○	○
Uplifted	○	○	○	○	○
Creative	○	○	○	○	○

Rating ☆ ☆ ☆ ☆ ☆

Strain _____

Grower _____   Date _____

Acquired _____ $ _____

THC % ____
CBD % ____

- [ ] Indica
- [ ] Sativa
- [ ] Hybrid

- [ ] Flower
- [ ] Edible
- [ ] Concentrate

Try again?
- [ ] Yes
- [ ] No

- [ ] Smoked
  - [ ] Rolled
  - [ ] Pipe
- [ ] Ate
- [ ] Dabbed
- [ ] Vaped

Symptoms Relieved

_____

_____

_____

_____

_____

Sweet

Fruity   Floral

Sour   Spicy

Earthy   Herbal

Woodsy

Notes

_____

_____

_____

_____

_____

_____

Effects	Strength				
Peaceful	○	○	○	○	○
Sleepy	○	○	○	○	○
Pain Relief	○	○	○	○	○
Hungry	○	○	○	○	○
Uplifted	○	○	○	○	○
Creative	○	○	○	○	○

Rating ☆ ☆ ☆ ☆ ☆

Strain _____

Grower _____ Date _____

Acquired _____ $ _____

THC % ____
CBD % ____

- [ ] Indica
- [ ] Sativa
- [ ] Hybrid

- [ ] Flower
- [ ] Edible
- [ ] Concentrate

Try again?
- [ ] Yes
- [ ] No

- [ ] Smoked
  - [ ] Rolled
  - [ ] Pipe
- [ ] Ate
- [ ] Dabbed
- [ ] Vaped

Symptoms Relieved

_____

_____

_____

_____

_____

Sweet

Fruity   Floral

Sour   Spicy

Earthy   Herbal

Woodsy

Notes

_____

_____

_____

_____

_____

_____

Effects	Strength				
Peaceful	○	○	○	○	○
Sleepy	○	○	○	○	○
Pain Relief	○	○	○	○	○
Hungry	○	○	○	○	○
Uplifted	○	○	○	○	○
Creative	○	○	○	○	○

Rating ☆ ☆ ☆ ☆ ☆

Strain _____

Grower _____ Date _____

Acquired _____ $ _____

THC % ___	☐ Indica	☐ Flower	Try again?
CBD % ___	☐ Sativa	☐ Edible	☐ Yes
	☐ Hybrid	☐ Concentrate	☐ No

☐ Smoked   ☐ Ate
  ☐ Rolled   ☐ Dabbed
  ☐ Pipe   ☐ Vaped

Symptoms Relieved

_____

_____

_____

_____

_____

Sweet
Fruity   Floral
Sour   Spicy
Earthy   Herbal
Woodsy

Notes

_____

_____

_____

_____

_____

_____

Effects	Strength
Peaceful	○ ○ ○ ○ ○
Sleepy	○ ○ ○ ○ ○
Pain Relief	○ ○ ○ ○ ○
Hungry	○ ○ ○ ○ ○
Uplifted	○ ○ ○ ○ ○
Creative	○ ○ ○ ○ ○

Rating ☆ ☆ ☆ ☆ ☆

Strain _____

Grower _____   Date _____

Acquired _____ $ _____

THC % ____
CBD % ____

- [ ] Indica
- [ ] Sativa
- [ ] Hybrid

- [ ] Flower
- [ ] Edible
- [ ] Concentrate

Try again?
- [ ] Yes
- [ ] No

- [ ] Smoked
  - [ ] Rolled
  - [ ] Pipe
- [ ] Ate
- [ ] Dabbed
- [ ] Vaped

Symptoms Relieved

_____

_____

_____

_____

_____

Notes

_____

_____

_____

_____

_____

_____

Sweet

Fruity   Floral

Sour   Spicy

Earthy   Herbal

Woodsy

Effects	Strength				
Peaceful	○	○	○	○	○
Sleepy	○	○	○	○	○
Pain Relief	○	○	○	○	○
Hungry	○	○	○	○	○
Uplifted	○	○	○	○	○
Creative	○	○	○	○	○

Rating ☆ ☆ ☆ ☆ ☆

Strain

Grower _____ Date _____

Acquired _____ $ _____

THC % ____
CBD % ____

- [ ] Indica
- [ ] Sativa
- [ ] Hybrid

- [ ] Flower
- [ ] Edible
- [ ] Concentrate

Try again?
- [ ] Yes
- [ ] No

- [ ] Smoked
  - [ ] Rolled
  - [ ] Pipe
- [ ] Ate
- [ ] Dabbed
- [ ] Vaped

Symptoms Relieved

_____

_____

_____

_____

_____

Notes

_____

_____

_____

_____

_____

_____

Sweet

Fruity   Floral

Sour   Spicy

Earthy   Herbal

Woodsy

Effects	Strength				
Peaceful	○	○	○	○	○
Sleepy	○	○	○	○	○
Pain Relief	○	○	○	○	○
Hungry	○	○	○	○	○
Uplifted	○	○	○	○	○
Creative	○	○	○	○	○

Rating ☆ ☆ ☆ ☆ ☆

Strain _____

Grower _____   Date _____

Acquired _____ $ _____

THC % ____	☐ Indica	☐ Flower	Try again?
CBD % ____	☐ Sativa	☐ Edible	☐ Yes
	☐ Hybrid	☐ Concentrate	☐ No

☐ Smoked   ☐ Ate
  ☐ Rolled   ☐ Dabbed
  ☐ Pipe   ☐ Vaped

Sweet

Fruity   Floral

Sour   Spicy

Symptoms Relieved

_____

_____   Earthy   Herbal

_____

_____   Woodsy

_____

Effects	Strength
Peaceful	○ ○ ○ ○ ○
Sleepy	○ ○ ○ ○ ○
Pain Relief	○ ○ ○ ○ ○
Hungry	○ ○ ○ ○ ○
Uplifted	○ ○ ○ ○ ○
Creative	○ ○ ○ ○ ○

Notes

_____

_____

_____

_____

_____   Rating ☆ ☆ ☆ ☆ ☆

_____

Strain

Grower _____ Date _____

Acquired _____ $ _____

THC % ___	☐ Indica	☐ Flower	Try again?
CBD % ___	☐ Sativa	☐ Edible	☐ Yes
	☐ Hybrid	☐ Concentrate	☐ No

☐ Smoked   ☐ Ate
   ☐ Rolled   ☐ Dabbed
   ☐ Pipe   ☐ Vaped

Symptoms Relieved

_____

_____

_____

_____

Notes

_____

_____

_____

_____

_____

_____

Sweet

Fruity   Floral

Sour   Spicy

Earthy   Herbal

Woodsy

Effects	Strength
Peaceful	○ ○ ○ ○ ○
Sleepy	○ ○ ○ ○ ○
Pain Relief	○ ○ ○ ○ ○
Hungry	○ ○ ○ ○ ○
Uplifted	○ ○ ○ ○ ○
Creative	○ ○ ○ ○ ○

Rating ☆ ☆ ☆ ☆ ☆

Strain _____

Grower _____ Date _____

Acquired _____ $ _____

THC % ____	☐ Indica	☐ Flower	Try again?
CBD % ____	☐ Sativa	☐ Edible	☐ Yes
	☐ Hybrid	☐ Concentrate	☐ No

☐ Smoked ☐ Ate
  ☐ Rolled ☐ Dabbed
  ☐ Pipe ☐ Vaped

Symptoms Relieved

_____

_____

_____

_____

_____

Notes

_____

_____

_____

_____

_____

_____

Sweet

Fruity   Floral

Sour   Spicy

Earthy   Herbal

Woodsy

Effects	Strength				
Peaceful	○	○	○	○	○
Sleepy	○	○	○	○	○
Pain Relief	○	○	○	○	○
Hungry	○	○	○	○	○
Uplifted	○	○	○	○	○
Creative	○	○	○	○	○

Rating ☆ ☆ ☆ ☆ ☆

Strain

Grower _____ Date _____

Acquired _____ $ _____

THC % ____
CBD % ____

- [ ] Indica
- [ ] Sativa
- [ ] Hybrid

- [ ] Flower
- [ ] Edible
- [ ] Concentrate

Try again?
- [ ] Yes
- [ ] No

- [ ] Smoked
  - [ ] Rolled
  - [ ] Pipe
- [ ] Ate
- [ ] Dabbed
- [ ] Vaped

Symptoms Relieved

_____

_____

_____

_____

_____

Sweet / Floral / Spicy / Herbal / Woodsy / Earthy / Sour / Fruity

Notes

_____

_____

_____

_____

_____

_____

Effects	Strength				
Peaceful	○	○	○	○	○
Sleepy	○	○	○	○	○
Pain Relief	○	○	○	○	○
Hungry	○	○	○	○	○
Uplifted	○	○	○	○	○
Creative	○	○	○	○	○

Rating ☆ ☆ ☆ ☆ ☆

Strain _____

Grower _____   Date _____

Acquired _____ $ _____

THC % ____
CBD % ____

- [ ] Indica
- [ ] Sativa
- [ ] Hybrid

- [ ] Flower
- [ ] Edible
- [ ] Concentrate

Try again?
- [ ] Yes
- [ ] No

- [ ] Smoked
  - [ ] Rolled
  - [ ] Pipe
- [ ] Ate
- [ ] Dabbed
- [ ] Vaped

Symptoms Relieved

_____

_____

_____

_____

_____

Sweet

Fruity   Floral

Sour   Spicy

Earthy   Herbal

Woodsy

Notes

_____

_____

_____

_____

_____

_____

Effects	Strength				
Peaceful	○	○	○	○	○
Sleepy	○	○	○	○	○
Pain Relief	○	○	○	○	○
Hungry	○	○	○	○	○
Uplifted	○	○	○	○	○
Creative	○	○	○	○	○

Rating ☆ ☆ ☆ ☆ ☆

Strain

Grower _____ Date _____

Acquired _____ $ _____

THC % ____	☐ Indica
	☐ Sativa
CBD % ____	☐ Hybrid

☐ Flower
☐ Edible
☐ Concentrate

Try again?
☐ Yes
☐ No

☐ Smoked   ☐ Ate
　☐ Rolled   ☐ Dabbed
　☐ Pipe   ☐ Vaped

Sweet
Fruity　　　　　　　Floral
Sour　　　　　　　　Spicy
Earthy　　　　　　　Herbal
Woodsy

Symptoms Relieved

_____
_____
_____
_____
_____

Notes

_____
_____
_____
_____
_____
_____

Effects	Strength
Peaceful	○ ○ ○ ○ ○
Sleepy	○ ○ ○ ○ ○
Pain Relief	○ ○ ○ ○ ○
Hungry	○ ○ ○ ○ ○
Uplifted	○ ○ ○ ○ ○
Creative	○ ○ ○ ○ ○

Rating ☆ ☆ ☆ ☆ ☆

Strain _____

Grower _____   Date _____

Acquired _____ $ _____

THC % ___	☐ Indica
CBD % ___	☐ Sativa
	☐ Hybrid

☐ Flower
☐ Edible
☐ Concentrate

Try again?
☐ Yes
☐ No

☐ Smoked   ☐ Ate
  ☐ Rolled   ☐ Dabbed
  ☐ Pipe   ☐ Vaped

Symptoms Relieved

_____

_____

_____

_____

Notes

_____

_____

_____

_____

_____

Sweet
Fruity   Floral
Sour   Spicy
Earthy   Herbal
Woodsy

Effects	Strength
Peaceful	○ ○ ○ ○ ○
Sleepy	○ ○ ○ ○ ○
Pain Relief	○ ○ ○ ○ ○
Hungry	○ ○ ○ ○ ○
Uplifted	○ ○ ○ ○ ○
Creative	○ ○ ○ ○ ○

Rating ☆ ☆ ☆ ☆ ☆

Strain

Grower _____   Date _____

Acquired _____ $ _____

THC % ____ CBD % ____	☐ Indica ☐ Sativa ☐ Hybrid	☐ Flower ☐ Edible ☐ Concentrate	Try again? ☐ Yes ☐ No

☐ Smoked   ☐ Ate
   ☐ Rolled   ☐ Dabbed
   ☐ Pipe   ☐ Vaped

Symptoms Relieved

_____
_____
_____
_____
_____

Notes

_____
_____
_____
_____
_____
_____

Sweet

Fruity   Floral

Sour   Spicy

Earthy   Herbal

Woodsy

Effects	Strength
Peaceful	○ ○ ○ ○ ○
Sleepy	○ ○ ○ ○ ○
Pain Relief	○ ○ ○ ○ ○
Hungry	○ ○ ○ ○ ○
Uplifted	○ ○ ○ ○ ○
Creative	○ ○ ○ ○ ○

Rating ☆ ☆ ☆ ☆ ☆

Strain _____

Grower _____ Date _____

Acquired _____ $ _____

THC % ____ CBD % ____	☐ Indica ☐ Sativa ☐ Hybrid	☐ Flower ☐ Edible ☐ Concentrate	Try again? ☐ Yes ☐ No

☐ Smoked ☐ Ate
  ☐ Rolled ☐ Dabbed
  ☐ Pipe ☐ Vaped

Symptoms Relieved

_____

_____

_____

_____

Notes

_____

_____

_____

_____

_____

_____

Sweet

Fruity   Floral

Sour   Spicy

Earthy   Herbal

Woodsy

Effects	Strength
Peaceful	○ ○ ○ ○ ○
Sleepy	○ ○ ○ ○ ○
Pain Relief	○ ○ ○ ○ ○
Hungry	○ ○ ○ ○ ○
Uplifted	○ ○ ○ ○ ○
Creative	○ ○ ○ ○ ○

Rating ☆ ☆ ☆ ☆ ☆

Strain

Grower _____ Date _____

Acquired _____ $ _____

THC % ____
CBD % ____

- [ ] Indica
- [ ] Sativa
- [ ] Hybrid

- [ ] Flower
- [ ] Edible
- [ ] Concentrate

Try again?
- [ ] Yes
- [ ] No

- [ ] Smoked
  - [ ] Rolled
  - [ ] Pipe
- [ ] Ate
- [ ] Dabbed
- [ ] Vaped

Symptoms Relieved

_____

_____

_____

_____

_____

Sweet
Fruity
Floral
Sour
Spicy
Earthy
Herbal
Woodsy

Notes

_____

_____

_____

_____

_____

_____

Effects	Strength				
Peaceful	○	○	○	○	○
Sleepy	○	○	○	○	○
Pain Relief	○	○	○	○	○
Hungry	○	○	○	○	○
Uplifted	○	○	○	○	○
Creative	○	○	○	○	○

Rating ☆ ☆ ☆ ☆ ☆

Strain _____

Grower _____ Date _____

Acquired _____ $ _____

THC % ____	☐ Indica
CBD % ____	☐ Sativa
	☐ Hybrid

☐ Flower	
☐ Edible	
☐ Concentrate	

Try again?
☐ Yes
☐ No

☐ Smoked ☐ Ate
☐ Rolled ☐ Dabbed
☐ Pipe ☐ Vaped

Symptoms Relieved

_____

_____

_____

_____

_____

Notes

_____

_____

_____

_____

_____

_____

Sweet

Fruity   Floral

Sour   Spicy

Earthy   Herbal

Woodsy

Effects	Strength
Peaceful	○ ○ ○ ○ ○
Sleepy	○ ○ ○ ○ ○
Pain Relief	○ ○ ○ ○ ○
Hungry	○ ○ ○ ○ ○
Uplifted	○ ○ ○ ○ ○
Creative	○ ○ ○ ○ ○

Rating ☆ ☆ ☆ ☆ ☆

Strain

Grower _____ Date _____

Acquired _____ $ _____

THC % _____
CBD % _____

- [ ] Indica
- [ ] Sativa
- [ ] Hybrid

- [ ] Flower
- [ ] Edible
- [ ] Concentrate

Try again?
- [ ] Yes
- [ ] No

- [ ] Smoked
  - [ ] Rolled
  - [ ] Pipe
- [ ] Ate
- [ ] Dabbed
- [ ] Vaped

Symptoms Relieved

_____

_____

_____

_____

_____

Notes

_____

_____

_____

_____

_____

Sweet
Fruity   Floral
Sour   Spicy
Earthy   Herbal
Woodsy

Effects	Strength				
Peaceful	○	○	○	○	○
Sleepy	○	○	○	○	○
Pain Relief	○	○	○	○	○
Hungry	○	○	○	○	○
Uplifted	○	○	○	○	○
Creative	○	○	○	○	○

Rating ☆ ☆ ☆ ☆ ☆

Strain _____

Grower _____ Date _____

Acquired _____ $ _____

THC % ___	☐ Indica	☐ Flower	Try again?
CBD % ___	☐ Sativa	☐ Edible	☐ Yes
	☐ Hybrid	☐ Concentrate	☐ No

☐ Smoked   ☐ Ate
  ☐ Rolled   ☐ Dabbed
  ☐ Pipe   ☐ Vaped

Sweet

Fruity   Floral

Sour   Spicy

Symptoms Relieved

Earthy   Herbal

_____

_____

Woodsy

_____

_____

Effects	Strength
Peaceful	○ ○ ○ ○ ○
Sleepy	○ ○ ○ ○ ○
Pain Relief	○ ○ ○ ○ ○
Hungry	○ ○ ○ ○ ○
Uplifted	○ ○ ○ ○ ○
Creative	○ ○ ○ ○ ○

Notes

_____

_____

_____

_____

Rating ☆ ☆ ☆ ☆ ☆

_____

Strain

Grower _____   Date _____

Acquired _____ $ _____

THC % ___
CBD % ___

☐ Indica
☐ Sativa
☐ Hybrid

☐ Flower
☐ Edible
☐ Concentrate

Try again?
☐ Yes
☐ No

☐ Smoked
　☐ Rolled
　☐ Pipe

☐ Ate
☐ Dabbed
☐ Vaped

Symptoms Relieved

_____

_____

_____

_____

_____

Sweet

Fruity

Floral

Sour

Spicy

Earthy

Herbal

Woodsy

Notes

_____

_____

_____

_____

_____

_____

Effects	Strength				
Peaceful	○	○	○	○	○
Sleepy	○	○	○	○	○
Pain Relief	○	○	○	○	○
Hungry	○	○	○	○	○
Uplifted	○	○	○	○	○
Creative	○	○	○	○	○

Rating ☆ ☆ ☆ ☆ ☆

Strain

Grower _____ Date _____

Acquired _____ $ _____

THC % ____	☐ Indica	☐ Flower	Try again?
CBD % ____	☐ Sativa	☐ Edible	☐ Yes
	☐ Hybrid	☐ Concentrate	☐ No

☐ Smoked ☐ Ate
   ☐ Rolled ☐ Dabbed
   ☐ Pipe ☐ Vaped

Symptoms Relieved

_____

_____

_____

_____

_____

Sweet

Fruity   Floral

Sour   Spicy

Earthy   Herbal

Woodsy

Notes

_____

_____

_____

_____

_____

_____

Effects	Strength				
Peaceful	○	○	○	○	○
Sleepy	○	○	○	○	○
Pain Relief	○	○	○	○	○
Hungry	○	○	○	○	○
Uplifted	○	○	○	○	○
Creative	○	○	○	○	○

Rating ☆ ☆ ☆ ☆ ☆

Strain _____

Grower _____   Date _____

Acquired _____ $ _____

THC % ____	☐ Indica	☐ Flower	Try again?
CBD % ____	☐ Sativa	☐ Edible	☐ Yes
	☐ Hybrid	☐ Concentrate	☐ No

☐ Smoked   ☐ Ate
  ☐ Rolled   ☐ Dabbed
  ☐ Pipe   ☐ Vaped

Symptoms Relieved

_____

_____

_____

_____

_____

Sweet

Fruity   Floral

Sour   Spicy

Earthy   Herbal

Woodsy

Notes

_____

_____

_____

_____

_____

_____

Effects	Strength
Peaceful	○ ○ ○ ○ ○
Sleepy	○ ○ ○ ○ ○
Pain Relief	○ ○ ○ ○ ○
Hungry	○ ○ ○ ○ ○
Uplifted	○ ○ ○ ○ ○
Creative	○ ○ ○ ○ ○

Rating ☆ ☆ ☆ ☆ ☆

Strain _____

Grower _____   Date _____

Acquired _____ $ _____

THC % ____ CBD % ____	☐ Indica ☐ Sativa ☐ Hybrid	☐ Flower ☐ Edible ☐ Concentrate	Try again? ☐ Yes ☐ No

☐ Smoked   ☐ Ate
   ☐ Rolled   ☐ Dabbed
   ☐ Pipe   ☐ Vaped

Symptoms Relieved

_____

_____

_____

_____

_____

Notes

_____

_____

_____

_____

_____

_____

Sweet

Fruity   Floral

Sour   Spicy

Earthy   Herbal

Woodsy

Effects	Strength				
Peaceful	○	○	○	○	○
Sleepy	○	○	○	○	○
Pain Relief	○	○	○	○	○
Hungry	○	○	○	○	○
Uplifted	○	○	○	○	○
Creative	○	○	○	○	○

Rating ☆ ☆ ☆ ☆ ☆

Strain

Grower _____   Date _____

Acquired _____ $ _____

THC % ____	☐ Indica	☐ Flower	Try again?
CBD % ____	☐ Sativa	☐ Edible	☐ Yes
	☐ Hybrid	☐ Concentrate	☐ No

☐ Smoked   ☐ Ate
  ☐ Rolled   ☐ Dabbed
  ☐ Pipe   ☐ Vaped

Symptoms Relieved

_____

_____

_____

_____

_____

Sweet

Fruity   Floral

Sour   Spicy

Earthy   Herbal

Woodsy

Notes

_____

_____

_____

_____

_____

Effects	Strength
Peaceful	○ ○ ○ ○ ○
Sleepy	○ ○ ○ ○ ○
Pain Relief	○ ○ ○ ○ ○
Hungry	○ ○ ○ ○ ○
Uplifted	○ ○ ○ ○ ○
Creative	○ ○ ○ ○ ○

Rating ☆ ☆ ☆ ☆ ☆

Strain _____

Grower _____ Date _____

Acquired _____ $ _____

THC % ____	☐ Indica	☐ Flower	Try again?
CBD % ____	☐ Sativa	☐ Edible	☐ Yes
	☐ Hybrid	☐ Concentrate	☐ No

☐ Smoked   ☐ Ate
  ☐ Rolled   ☐ Dabbed
  ☐ Pipe   ☐ Vaped

Symptoms Relieved

_____
_____
_____
_____
_____

Notes

_____
_____
_____
_____
_____
_____

Sweet

Fruity   Floral

Sour   Spicy

Earthy   Herbal

Woodsy

Effects	Strength
Peaceful	○ ○ ○ ○ ○
Sleepy	○ ○ ○ ○ ○
Pain Relief	○ ○ ○ ○ ○
Hungry	○ ○ ○ ○ ○
Uplifted	○ ○ ○ ○ ○
Creative	○ ○ ○ ○ ○

Rating ☆ ☆ ☆ ☆ ☆

Strain

Grower _____ Date _____

Acquired _____ $ _____

THC % ___	☐ Indica	☐ Flower	Try again?
CBD % ___	☐ Sativa	☐ Edible	☐ Yes
	☐ Hybrid	☐ Concentrate	☐ No

☐ Smoked   ☐ Ate
   ☐ Rolled   ☐ Dabbed
   ☐ Pipe   ☐ Vaped

Symptoms Relieved

_____

_____

_____

_____

_____

Sweet
Fruity   Floral
Sour   Spicy
Earthy   Herbal
Woodsy

Notes

_____

_____

_____

_____

_____

_____

_____

Effects	Strength
Peaceful	○ ○ ○ ○ ○
Sleepy	○ ○ ○ ○ ○
Pain Relief	○ ○ ○ ○ ○
Hungry	○ ○ ○ ○ ○
Uplifted	○ ○ ○ ○ ○
Creative	○ ○ ○ ○ ○

Rating ☆ ☆ ☆ ☆ ☆

Strain _____

Grower _____ Date _____

Acquired _____ $ _____

THC % ____	☐ Indica	☐ Flower	Try again?
CBD % ____	☐ Sativa	☐ Edible	☐ Yes
	☐ Hybrid	☐ Concentrate	☐ No

☐ Smoked   ☐ Ate
  ☐ Rolled   ☐ Dabbed
  ☐ Pipe   ☐ Vaped

Sweet

Fruity   Floral

Sour   Spicy

Symptoms Relieved

_____

_____   Earthy   Herbal

_____   Woodsy

_____

_____

Effects	Strength _____

Notes

Peaceful	○	○	○	○	○
Sleepy	○	○	○	○	○
Pain Relief	○	○	○	○	○
Hungry	○	○	○	○	○
Uplifted	○	○	○	○	○
Creative	○	○	○	○	○

_____

_____

_____

_____

_____

Rating ☆ ☆ ☆ ☆ ☆

_____

Strain _____

Grower _____   Date _____

Acquired _____ $ _____

THC % ____   ☐ Indica   ☐ Flower   Try again?
                ☐ Sativa   ☐ Edible   ☐ Yes
CBD % ____   ☐ Hybrid   ☐ Concentrate   ☐ No

☐ Smoked   ☐ Ate
  ☐ Rolled   ☐ Dabbed
  ☐ Pipe   ☐ Vaped

Symptoms Relieved

_____

_____

_____

_____

_____

Notes

_____

_____

_____

_____

_____

_____

Effects	Strength				
Peaceful	○	○	○	○	○
Sleepy	○	○	○	○	○
Pain Relief	○	○	○	○	○
Hungry	○	○	○	○	○
Uplifted	○	○	○	○	○
Creative	○	○	○	○	○

Rating ☆ ☆ ☆ ☆ ☆

Strain _____

Grower _____ Date _____

Acquired _____ $ _____

THC % ____ CBD % ____	☐ Indica ☐ Sativa ☐ Hybrid	☐ Flower ☐ Edible ☐ Concentrate	Try again? ☐ Yes ☐ No

☐ Smoked   ☐ Ate
  ☐ Rolled   ☐ Dabbed
  ☐ Pipe   ☐ Vaped

Symptoms Relieved

_____

_____

_____

_____

_____

Notes

_____

_____

_____

_____

_____

_____

Sweet
Fruity   Floral
Sour   Spicy
Earthy   Herbal
Woodsy

Effects	Strength				
Peaceful	○	○	○	○	○
Sleepy	○	○	○	○	○
Pain Relief	○	○	○	○	○
Hungry	○	○	○	○	○
Uplifted	○	○	○	○	○
Creative	○	○	○	○	○

Rating ☆ ☆ ☆ ☆ ☆

Strain _____

Grower _____   Date _____

Acquired _____ $ _____

THC % ____	☐ Indica ☐ Sativa ☐ Hybrid	☐ Flower ☐ Edible ☐ Concentrate	Try again? ☐ Yes ☐ No
CBD % ____			

☐ Smoked   ☐ Ate
  ☐ Rolled   ☐ Dabbed
  ☐ Pipe   ☐ Vaped

Symptoms Relieved

_____
_____
_____
_____
_____

Notes

_____
_____
_____
_____
_____
_____

Sweet
Fruity
Floral
Sour
Spicy
Earthy
Herbal
Woodsy

Effects	Strength
Peaceful	○ ○ ○ ○ ○
Sleepy	○ ○ ○ ○ ○
Pain Relief	○ ○ ○ ○ ○
Hungry	○ ○ ○ ○ ○
Uplifted	○ ○ ○ ○ ○
Creative	○ ○ ○ ○ ○

Rating ☆ ☆ ☆ ☆ ☆

Strain _____

Grower _____   Date _____

Acquired _____ $ _____

THC % ____	☐ Indica	☐ Flower	Try again?
CBD % ____	☐ Sativa	☐ Edible	☐ Yes
	☐ Hybrid	☐ Concentrate	☐ No

☐ Smoked   ☐ Ate
  ☐ Rolled   ☐ Dabbed
  ☐ Pipe   ☐ Vaped

Sweet

Fruity   Floral

Symptoms Relieved

Sour   Spicy

_____

_____

_____   Earthy   Herbal

_____

Woodsy

Effects	Strength				
Peaceful	○	○	○	○	○
Notes
| Sleepy | ○ | ○ | ○ | ○ | ○ |
| Pain Relief | ○ | ○ | ○ | ○ | ○ |
_____
| Hungry | ○ | ○ | ○ | ○ | ○ |
_____
| Uplifted | ○ | ○ | ○ | ○ | ○ |
_____
| Creative | ○ | ○ | ○ | ○ | ○ |
_____

_____

Rating ☆ ☆ ☆ ☆ ☆

_____

Strain _____

Grower _____ Date _____

Acquired _____ $ _____

THC % ____ CBD % ____	☐ Indica ☐ Sativa ☐ Hybrid	☐ Flower ☐ Edible ☐ Concentrate	Try again? ☐ Yes ☐ No

☐ Smoked   ☐ Ate
   ☐ Rolled   ☐ Dabbed
   ☐ Pipe   ☐ Vaped

Symptoms Relieved

_____
_____
_____
_____
_____

Sweet
Fruity
Floral
Sour
Spicy
Earthy
Herbal
Woodsy

Notes

_____
_____
_____
_____
_____
_____
_____

Effects	Strength				
Peaceful	○	○	○	○	○
Sleepy	○	○	○	○	○
Pain Relief	○	○	○	○	○
Hungry	○	○	○	○	○
Uplifted	○	○	○	○	○
Creative	○	○	○	○	○

Rating ☆ ☆ ☆ ☆ ☆

Strain _____

Grower _____   Date _____

Acquired _____ $ _____

THC % ____
CBD % ____

☐ Indica
☐ Sativa
☐ Hybrid

☐ Flower
☐ Edible
☐ Concentrate

Try again?
☐ Yes
☐ No

☐ Smoked
  ☐ Rolled
  ☐ Pipe

☐ Ate
☐ Dabbed
☐ Vaped

Sweet

Fruity   Floral

Symptoms Relieved

Sour   Spicy

_____

_____

_____   Earthy   Herbal

_____

_____   Woodsy

Effects	Strength				
Peaceful	○	○	○	○	○
Sleepy	○	○	○	○	○

Notes

Pain Relief	○	○	○	○	○
Hungry	○	○	○	○	○
Uplifted	○	○	○	○	○
Creative	○	○	○	○	○

_____

_____

_____

_____

Rating ☆ ☆ ☆ ☆ ☆

_____

_____

Strain _____

Grower _____ Date _____

Acquired _____ $ _____

THC % ____	☐ Indica	☐ Flower	Try again?
CBD % ____	☐ Sativa	☐ Edible	☐ Yes
	☐ Hybrid	☐ Concentrate	☐ No

☐ Smoked   ☐ Ate
  ☐ Rolled   ☐ Dabbed
  ☐ Pipe   ☐ Vaped

Symptoms Relieved

_____

_____

_____

_____

_____

Notes

_____

_____

_____

_____

_____

_____

_____

Sweet
Fruity / Floral
Sour / Spicy
Earthy / Herbal
Woodsy

Effects	Strength
Peaceful	○ ○ ○ ○ ○
Sleepy	○ ○ ○ ○ ○
Pain Relief	○ ○ ○ ○ ○
Hungry	○ ○ ○ ○ ○
Uplifted	○ ○ ○ ○ ○
Creative	○ ○ ○ ○ ○

Rating ☆ ☆ ☆ ☆ ☆

Strain _____

Grower _____ Date _____

Acquired _____ $ _____

THC % ___	☐ Indica
CBD % ___	☐ Sativa
	☐ Hybrid

☐ Flower ☐ Edible ☐ Concentrate

Try again?
☐ Yes
☐ No

☐ Smoked   ☐ Ate
  ☐ Rolled   ☐ Dabbed
  ☐ Pipe   ☐ Vaped

Symptoms Relieved

_____

_____

_____

_____

_____

Sweet
Fruity   Floral
Sour   Spicy
Earthy   Herbal
Woodsy

Notes

_____

_____

_____

_____

_____

Effects	Strength
Peaceful	○ ○ ○ ○ ○
Sleepy	○ ○ ○ ○ ○
Pain Relief	○ ○ ○ ○ ○
Hungry	○ ○ ○ ○ ○
Uplifted	○ ○ ○ ○ ○
Creative	○ ○ ○ ○ ○

Rating ☆ ☆ ☆ ☆ ☆

Strain _____

Grower _____ Date _____

Acquired _____ $ _____

THC % ____ CBD % ____	☐ Indica ☐ Sativa ☐ Hybrid	☐ Flower ☐ Edible ☐ Concentrate	Try again? ☐ Yes ☐ No

☐ Smoked   ☐ Ate
   ☐ Rolled   ☐ Dabbed
   ☐ Pipe   ☐ Vaped

Symptoms Relieved

_____

_____

_____

_____

_____

Sweet

Fruity   Floral

Sour   Spicy

Earthy   Herbal

Woodsy

Effects	Strength
Peaceful	○ ○ ○ ○ ○
Sleepy	○ ○ ○ ○ ○
Pain Relief	○ ○ ○ ○ ○
Hungry	○ ○ ○ ○ ○
Uplifted	○ ○ ○ ○ ○
Creative	○ ○ ○ ○ ○

Notes

_____

_____

_____

_____

_____

_____

Rating ☆ ☆ ☆ ☆ ☆

Strain _____

Grower _____ Date _____

Acquired _____ $ _____

THC % ____ CBD % ____	☐ Indica ☐ Sativa ☐ Hybrid	☐ Flower ☐ Edible ☐ Concentrate	Try again? ☐ Yes ☐ No

☐ Smoked   ☐ Ate
   ☐ Rolled   ☐ Dabbed
   ☐ Pipe   ☐ Vaped

Symptoms Relieved

_____

_____

_____

_____

_____

Notes

_____

_____

_____

_____

_____

_____

Sweet

Fruity   Floral

Sour   Spicy

Earthy   Herbal

Woodsy

Effects	Strength
Peaceful	○ ○ ○ ○ ○
Sleepy	○ ○ ○ ○ ○
Pain Relief	○ ○ ○ ○ ○
Hungry	○ ○ ○ ○ ○
Uplifted	○ ○ ○ ○ ○
Creative	○ ○ ○ ○ ○

Rating ☆ ☆ ☆ ☆ ☆

Strain

Grower _____   Date _____

Acquired _____ $ _____

THC % ____ CBD % ____	☐ Indica ☐ Sativa ☐ Hybrid

☐ Flower ☐ Edible ☐ Concentrate	Try again? ☐ Yes ☐ No

☐ Smoked   ☐ Ate
   ☐ Rolled   ☐ Dabbed
   ☐ Pipe   ☐ Vaped

Symptoms Relieved

_____

_____

_____

_____

Sweet
Fruity
Floral
Sour
Spicy
Earthy
Herbal
Woodsy

Notes

_____

_____

_____

_____

_____

_____

Effects	Strength
Peaceful	○ ○ ○ ○ ○
Sleepy	○ ○ ○ ○ ○
Pain Relief	○ ○ ○ ○ ○
Hungry	○ ○ ○ ○ ○
Uplifted	○ ○ ○ ○ ○
Creative	○ ○ ○ ○ ○

Rating ☆ ☆ ☆ ☆ ☆

Strain _____

Grower _____ Date _____

Acquired _____ $ _____

THC % ____
CBD % ____

- [ ] Indica
- [ ] Sativa
- [ ] Hybrid

- [ ] Flower
- [ ] Edible
- [ ] Concentrate

Try again?
- [ ] Yes
- [ ] No

- [ ] Smoked
  - [ ] Rolled
  - [ ] Pipe
- [ ] Ate
- [ ] Dabbed
- [ ] Vaped

Symptoms Relieved

_____

_____

_____

_____

_____

Sweet

Fruity

Floral

Sour

Spicy

Earthy

Herbal

Woodsy

Notes

_____

_____

_____

_____

_____

_____

Effects	Strength				
Peaceful	◯	◯	◯	◯	◯
Sleepy	◯	◯	◯	◯	◯
Pain Relief	◯	◯	◯	◯	◯
Hungry	◯	◯	◯	◯	◯
Uplifted	◯	◯	◯	◯	◯
Creative	◯	◯	◯	◯	◯

Rating ☆ ☆ ☆ ☆ ☆

Strain _____

Grower _____ Date _____

Acquired _____ $ _____

THC % ____
CBD % ____

☐ Indica
☐ Sativa
☐ Hybrid

☐ Flower
☐ Edible
☐ Concentrate

Try again?
☐ Yes
☐ No

☐ Smoked
  ☐ Rolled
  ☐ Pipe
☐ Ate
☐ Dabbed
☐ Vaped

Symptoms Relieved

_____

_____

_____

_____

_____

Sweet

Fruity

Floral

Sour

Spicy

Earthy

Herbal

Woodsy

Notes

_____

_____

_____

_____

_____

_____

Effects	Strength				
Peaceful	○	○	○	○	○
Sleepy	○	○	○	○	○
Pain Relief	○	○	○	○	○
Hungry	○	○	○	○	○
Uplifted	○	○	○	○	○
Creative	○	○	○	○	○

Rating ☆ ☆ ☆ ☆ ☆

Strain _____

Grower _____   Date _____

Acquired _____ $ _____

THC % ____ CBD % ____	☐ Indica ☐ Sativa ☐ Hybrid

☐ Flower ☐ Edible ☐ Concentrate	**Try again?** ☐ Yes ☐ No

☐ Smoked   ☐ Ate
   ☐ Rolled   ☐ Dabbed
   ☐ Pipe   ☐ Vaped

Symptoms Relieved

_____

_____

_____

_____

_____

Sweet

Fruity   Floral

Sour   Spicy

Earthy   Herbal

Woodsy

Effects	Strength
Peaceful	○ ○ ○ ○ ○
Sleepy	○ ○ ○ ○ ○
Pain Relief	○ ○ ○ ○ ○
Hungry	○ ○ ○ ○ ○
Uplifted	○ ○ ○ ○ ○
Creative	○ ○ ○ ○ ○

Notes

_____

_____

_____

_____

_____

_____

Rating ☆ ☆ ☆ ☆ ☆

Strain _____

Grower _____ Date _____

Acquired _____ $ _____

THC % ____
CBD % ____

- ☐ Indica
- ☐ Sativa
- ☐ Hybrid

- ☐ Flower
- ☐ Edible
- ☐ Concentrate

Try again?
- ☐ Yes
- ☐ No

- ☐ Smoked
  - ☐ Rolled
  - ☐ Pipe
- ☐ Ate
- ☐ Dabbed
- ☐ Vaped

Symptoms Relieved

_____

_____

_____

_____

_____

Sweet

Fruity

Floral

Sour

Spicy

Earthy

Herbal

Woodsy

Notes

_____

_____

_____

_____

_____

_____

Effects	Strength				
Peaceful	○	○	○	○	○
Sleepy	○	○	○	○	○
Pain Relief	○	○	○	○	○
Hungry	○	○	○	○	○
Uplifted	○	○	○	○	○
Creative	○	○	○	○	○

Rating ☆ ☆ ☆ ☆ ☆

Strain _____

Grower _____   Date _____

Acquired _____ $ _____

THC % ____	☐ Indica	☐ Flower	Try again?
CBD % ____	☐ Sativa	☐ Edible	☐ Yes
	☐ Hybrid	☐ Concentrate	☐ No

☐ Smoked   ☐ Ate
  ☐ Rolled   ☐ Dabbed
  ☐ Pipe   ☐ Vaped

Symptoms Relieved

_____

_____

_____

_____

_____

Sweet

Fruity   Floral

Sour   Spicy

Earthy   Herbal

Woodsy

Effects	Strength
Peaceful	○ ○ ○ ○ ○
Sleepy	○ ○ ○ ○ ○
Pain Relief	○ ○ ○ ○ ○
Hungry	○ ○ ○ ○ ○
Uplifted	○ ○ ○ ○ ○
Creative	○ ○ ○ ○ ○

Notes

_____

_____

_____

_____

_____

_____

_____

Rating ☆ ☆ ☆ ☆ ☆

Strain

Grower _____ Date _____

Acquired _____ $ _____

THC % ___	☐ Indica	☐ Flower	Try again?
CBD % ___	☐ Sativa	☐ Edible	☐ Yes
	☐ Hybrid	☐ Concentrate	☐ No

☐ Smoked   ☐ Ate
   ☐ Rolled   ☐ Dabbed
   ☐ Pipe   ☐ Vaped

Symptoms Relieved

_____

_____

_____

_____

Notes

_____

_____

_____

_____

_____

_____

Sweet

Fruity   Floral

Sour   Spicy

Earthy   Herbal

Woodsy

Effects	Strength
Peaceful	○ ○ ○ ○ ○
Sleepy	○ ○ ○ ○ ○
Pain Relief	○ ○ ○ ○ ○
Hungry	○ ○ ○ ○ ○
Uplifted	○ ○ ○ ○ ○
Creative	○ ○ ○ ○ ○

Rating ☆ ☆ ☆ ☆ ☆

Strain _____

Grower _____ Date _____

Acquired _____ $ _____

THC % ____
CBD % ____

☐ Indica
☐ Sativa
☐ Hybrid

☐ Flower
☐ Edible
☐ Concentrate

Try again?
☐ Yes
☐ No

☐ Smoked
  ☐ Rolled
  ☐ Pipe

☐ Ate
☐ Dabbed
☐ Vaped

Symptoms Relieved

_____

_____

_____

_____

_____

Notes

_____

_____

_____

_____

_____

_____

Sweet

Fruity

Floral

Sour

Spicy

Earthy

Herbal

Woodsy

Effects	Strength				
Peaceful	○	○	○	○	○
Sleepy	○	○	○	○	○
Pain Relief	○	○	○	○	○
Hungry	○	○	○	○	○
Uplifted	○	○	○	○	○
Creative	○	○	○	○	○

Rating ☆ ☆ ☆ ☆ ☆

Strain

Grower _____   Date _____

Acquired _____ $ _____

THC % ____	☐ Indica	☐ Flower	Try again?
CBD % ____	☐ Sativa	☐ Edible	☐ Yes
	☐ Hybrid	☐ Concentrate	☐ No

☐ Smoked   ☐ Ate
　☐ Rolled   ☐ Dabbed
　☐ Pipe   ☐ Vaped

Symptoms Relieved

_____

_____

_____

_____

_____

Notes

_____

_____

_____

_____

_____

_____

Sweet

Fruity   Floral

Sour   Spicy

Earthy   Herbal

Woodsy

Effects	Strength
Peaceful	○ ○ ○ ○ ○
Sleepy	○ ○ ○ ○ ○
Pain Relief	○ ○ ○ ○ ○
Hungry	○ ○ ○ ○ ○
Uplifted	○ ○ ○ ○ ○
Creative	○ ○ ○ ○ ○

Rating ☆ ☆ ☆ ☆ ☆

Strain _____

Grower _____   Date _____

Acquired _____ $ _____

THC % ___	☐ Indica	☐ Flower	Try again?
CBD % ___	☐ Sativa	☐ Edible	☐ Yes
	☐ Hybrid	☐ Concentrate	☐ No

☐ Smoked   ☐ Ate
  ☐ Rolled   ☐ Dabbed
  ☐ Pipe   ☐ Vaped

Symptoms Relieved

_____

_____

_____

_____

_____

Sweet

Fruity   Floral

Sour   Spicy

Earthy   Herbal

Woodsy

Notes

_____

_____

_____

_____

_____

_____

Effects	Strength
Peaceful	○ ○ ○ ○ ○
Sleepy	○ ○ ○ ○ ○
Pain Relief	○ ○ ○ ○ ○
Hungry	○ ○ ○ ○ ○
Uplifted	○ ○ ○ ○ ○
Creative	○ ○ ○ ○ ○

Rating ☆ ☆ ☆ ☆ ☆

Strain _____

Grower _____   Date _____

Acquired _____ $ _____

THC % ____	☐ Indica	☐ Flower	Try again?
CBD % ____	☐ Sativa	☐ Edible	☐ Yes
	☐ Hybrid	☐ Concentrate	☐ No

☐ Smoked   ☐ Ate
  ☐ Rolled   ☐ Dabbed
  ☐ Pipe   ☐ Vaped

Symptoms Relieved

_____

_____

_____

_____

_____

Sweet
Fruity   Floral
Sour   Spicy
Earthy   Herbal
Woodsy

Notes

_____

_____

_____

_____

_____

_____

_____

Effects	Strength
Peaceful	○ ○ ○ ○ ○
Sleepy	○ ○ ○ ○ ○
Pain Relief	○ ○ ○ ○ ○
Hungry	○ ○ ○ ○ ○
Uplifted	○ ○ ○ ○ ○
Creative	○ ○ ○ ○ ○

Rating ☆ ☆ ☆ ☆ ☆

Strain _____

Grower _____ Date _____

Acquired _____ $ _____

THC % ____	☐ Indica	☐ Flower	Try again?
CBD % ____	☐ Sativa	☐ Edible	☐ Yes
	☐ Hybrid	☐ Concentrate	☐ No

☐ Smoked ☐ Ate
  ☐ Rolled ☐ Dabbed
  ☐ Pipe ☐ Vaped

Symptoms Relieved

_____

_____

_____

_____

_____

Notes

_____

_____

_____

_____

_____

_____

_____

Sweet

Fruity   Floral

Sour   Spicy

Earthy   Herbal

Woodsy

Effects	Strength				
Peaceful	○	○	○	○	○
Sleepy	○	○	○	○	○
Pain Relief	○	○	○	○	○
Hungry	○	○	○	○	○
Uplifted	○	○	○	○	○
Creative	○	○	○	○	○

Rating ☆ ☆ ☆ ☆ ☆

Strain _____

Grower _____   Date _____

Acquired _____ $ _____

THC % ____	☐ Indica
	☐ Sativa
CBD % ____	☐ Hybrid

☐ Flower	☐ Edible
☐ Concentrate	

Try again?
☐ Yes
☐ No

☐ Smoked   ☐ Ate
  ☐ Rolled   ☐ Dabbed
  ☐ Pipe   ☐ Vaped

Symptoms Relieved

_____

_____

_____

_____

_____

Sweet

Fruity   Floral

Sour   Spicy

Earthy   Herbal

Woodsy

Notes

_____

_____

_____

_____

_____

_____

Effects	Strength				
Peaceful	○	○	○	○	○
Sleepy	○	○	○	○	○
Pain Relief	○	○	○	○	○
Hungry	○	○	○	○	○
Uplifted	○	○	○	○	○
Creative	○	○	○	○	○

Rating ☆ ☆ ☆ ☆ ☆

Strain _____

Grower _____   Date _____

Acquired _____ $ _____

THC % ____	☐ Indica	☐ Flower	Try again?
CBD % ____	☐ Sativa	☐ Edible	☐ Yes
	☐ Hybrid	☐ Concentrate	☐ No

☐ Smoked   ☐ Ate
  ☐ Rolled   ☐ Dabbed
  ☐ Pipe   ☐ Vaped

Symptoms Relieved

_____

_____

_____

_____

Sweet

Fruity   Floral

Sour   Spicy

Earthy   Herbal

Woodsy

Notes

_____

_____

_____

_____

_____

_____

Effects	Strength
Peaceful	○ ○ ○ ○ ○
Sleepy	○ ○ ○ ○ ○
Pain Relief	○ ○ ○ ○ ○
Hungry	○ ○ ○ ○ ○
Uplifted	○ ○ ○ ○ ○
Creative	○ ○ ○ ○ ○

Rating ☆ ☆ ☆ ☆ ☆

Strain _____

Grower _____   Date _____

Acquired _____ $ _____

| THC % ___ CBD % ___ | ☐ Indica ☐ Sativa ☐ Hybrid | ☐ Flower ☐ Edible ☐ Concentrate | Try again? ☐ Yes ☐ No |

☐ Smoked   ☐ Ate
  ☐ Rolled   ☐ Dabbed
  ☐ Pipe   ☐ Vaped

Symptoms Relieved

_____

_____

_____

_____

_____

Notes

_____

_____

_____

_____

_____

Sweet
Fruity   Floral
Sour   Spicy
Earthy   Herbal
Woodsy

Effects	Strength
Peaceful	○ ○ ○ ○ ○
Sleepy	○ ○ ○ ○ ○
Pain Relief	○ ○ ○ ○ ○
Hungry	○ ○ ○ ○ ○
Uplifted	○ ○ ○ ○ ○
Creative	○ ○ ○ ○ ○

Rating ☆ ☆ ☆ ☆ ☆

Strain _____

Grower _____ Date _____

Acquired _____ $ _____

THC % ____
CBD % ____

- [ ] Indica
- [ ] Sativa
- [ ] Hybrid

- [ ] Flower
- [ ] Edible
- [ ] Concentrate

Try again?
- [ ] Yes
- [ ] No

- [ ] Smoked
  - [ ] Rolled
  - [ ] Pipe
- [ ] Ate
- [ ] Dabbed
- [ ] Vaped

Symptoms Relieved

_____

_____

_____

_____

_____

Sweet

Fruity   Floral

Sour   Spicy

Earthy   Herbal

Woodsy

Notes

_____

_____

_____

_____

_____

_____

Effects	Strength				
Peaceful	○	○	○	○	○
Sleepy	○	○	○	○	○
Pain Relief	○	○	○	○	○
Hungry	○	○	○	○	○
Uplifted	○	○	○	○	○
Creative	○	○	○	○	○

Rating ☆ ☆ ☆ ☆ ☆

Strain

Grower _____ Date _____

Acquired _____ $ _____

| THC % ____
CBD % ____ | ☐ Indica
☐ Sativa
☐ Hybrid | ☐ Flower
☐ Edible
☐ Concentrate | Try again?
☐ Yes
☐ No |

☐ Smoked   ☐ Ate
  ☐ Rolled   ☐ Dabbed
  ☐ Pipe   ☐ Vaped

Symptoms Relieved

_____

_____

_____

_____

_____

Notes

_____

_____

_____

_____

_____

_____

Sweet

Fruity

Floral

Sour

Spicy

Earthy

Herbal

Woodsy

Effects	Strength				
Peaceful	○	○	○	○	○
Sleepy	○	○	○	○	○
Pain Relief	○	○	○	○	○
Hungry	○	○	○	○	○
Uplifted	○	○	○	○	○
Creative	○	○	○	○	○

Rating ☆ ☆ ☆ ☆ ☆

Strain _____

Grower _____   Date _____

Acquired _____ $ _____

THC % ____	☐ Indica	☐ Flower	Try again?
CBD % ____	☐ Sativa	☐ Edible	☐ Yes
	☐ Hybrid	☐ Concentrate	☐ No

☐ Smoked   ☐ Ate
  ☐ Rolled   ☐ Dabbed
  ☐ Pipe   ☐ Vaped

Symptoms Relieved

_____

_____

_____

_____

_____

Sweet
Fruity   Floral
Sour   Spicy
Earthy   Herbal
Woodsy

Notes

_____

_____

_____

_____

_____

_____

Effects	Strength				
Peaceful	○	○	○	○	○
Sleepy	○	○	○	○	○
Pain Relief	○	○	○	○	○
Hungry	○	○	○	○	○
Uplifted	○	○	○	○	○
Creative	○	○	○	○	○

Rating ☆ ☆ ☆ ☆ ☆

Strain _____

Grower _____ Date _____

Acquired _____ $ _____

THC % ___	☐ Indica	☐ Flower	Try again?
CBD % ___	☐ Sativa	☐ Edible	☐ Yes
	☐ Hybrid	☐ Concentrate	☐ No

☐ Smoked   ☐ Ate
  ☐ Rolled   ☐ Dabbed
  ☐ Pipe   ☐ Vaped

Symptoms Relieved

_____

_____

_____

_____

_____

Notes

_____

_____

_____

_____

_____

_____

_____

Sweet

Fruity   Floral

Sour   Spicy

Earthy   Herbal

Woodsy

Effects	Strength				
Peaceful	○	○	○	○	○
Sleepy	○	○	○	○	○
Pain Relief	○	○	○	○	○
Hungry	○	○	○	○	○
Uplifted	○	○	○	○	○
Creative	○	○	○	○	○

Rating ☆ ☆ ☆ ☆ ☆

Strain _____

Grower _____ Date _____

Acquired _____ $ _____

THC % ____	☐ Indica	☐ Flower	Try again?
CBD % ____	☐ Sativa	☐ Edible	☐ Yes
	☐ Hybrid	☐ Concentrate	☐ No

☐ Smoked   ☐ Ate
　☐ Rolled   ☐ Dabbed
　☐ Pipe   ☐ Vaped

Symptoms Relieved

_____

_____

_____

_____

_____

Sweet

Fruity   Floral

Sour   Spicy

Earthy   Herbal

Woodsy

Notes

_____

_____

_____

_____

_____

_____

Effects	Strength
Peaceful	○ ○ ○ ○ ○
Sleepy	○ ○ ○ ○ ○
Pain Relief	○ ○ ○ ○ ○
Hungry	○ ○ ○ ○ ○
Uplifted	○ ○ ○ ○ ○
Creative	○ ○ ○ ○ ○

Rating ☆ ☆ ☆ ☆ ☆

Strain _____

Grower _____ Date _____

Acquired _____ $ _____

THC % ___
CBD % ___

- [ ] Indica
- [ ] Sativa
- [ ] Hybrid

- [ ] Flower
- [ ] Edible
- [ ] Concentrate

Try again?
- [ ] Yes
- [ ] No

- [ ] Smoked
  - [ ] Rolled
  - [ ] Pipe
- [ ] Ate
- [ ] Dabbed
- [ ] Vaped

Symptoms Relieved

_____

_____

_____

_____

_____

Sweet

Fruity   Floral

Sour   Spicy

Earthy   Herbal

Woodsy

Notes

_____

_____

_____

_____

_____

_____

Effects	Strength				
Peaceful	○	○	○	○	○
Sleepy	○	○	○	○	○
Pain Relief	○	○	○	○	○
Hungry	○	○	○	○	○
Uplifted	○	○	○	○	○
Creative	○	○	○	○	○

Rating ☆ ☆ ☆ ☆ ☆

Strain _____

Grower _____ Date _____

Acquired _____ $ _____

THC % ___
CBD % ___

- [ ] Indica
- [ ] Sativa
- [ ] Hybrid

- [ ] Flower
- [ ] Edible
- [ ] Concentrate

Try again?
- [ ] Yes
- [ ] No

- [ ] Smoked
  - [ ] Rolled
  - [ ] Pipe
- [ ] Ate
- [ ] Dabbed
- [ ] Vaped

Symptoms Relieved

_____
_____
_____
_____
_____

Sweet
Fruity
Floral
Sour
Spicy
Earthy
Herbal
Woodsy

Notes

_____
_____
_____
_____
_____
_____

Effects	Strength				
Peaceful	○	○	○	○	○
Sleepy	○	○	○	○	○
Pain Relief	○	○	○	○	○
Hungry	○	○	○	○	○
Uplifted	○	○	○	○	○
Creative	○	○	○	○	○

Rating ☆ ☆ ☆ ☆ ☆

Strain

Grower _____ Date _____

Acquired _____ $ _____

THC % ____
CBD % ____

- [ ] Indica
- [ ] Sativa
- [ ] Hybrid

- [ ] Flower
- [ ] Edible
- [ ] Concentrate

Try again?
- [ ] Yes
- [ ] No

- [ ] Smoked
  - [ ] Rolled
  - [ ] Pipe
- [ ] Ate
- [ ] Dabbed
- [ ] Vaped

Symptoms Relieved

_____

_____

_____

_____

Sweet

Fruity   Floral

Sour   Spicy

Earthy   Herbal

Woodsy

Notes

_____

_____

_____

_____

_____

_____

Effects	Strength				
Peaceful	○	○	○	○	○
Sleepy	○	○	○	○	○
Pain Relief	○	○	○	○	○
Hungry	○	○	○	○	○
Uplifted	○	○	○	○	○
Creative	○	○	○	○	○

Rating ☆ ☆ ☆ ☆ ☆

Strain _____

Grower _____   Date _____

Acquired _____ $ _____

THC % ___	☐ Indica	☐ Flower	Try again?
CBD % ___	☐ Sativa	☐ Edible	☐ Yes
	☐ Hybrid	☐ Concentrate	☐ No

☐ Smoked   ☐ Ate
  ☐ Rolled   ☐ Dabbed
  ☐ Pipe   ☐ Vaped

Symptoms Relieved

_____

_____

_____

_____

_____

Sweet

Fruity   Floral

Sour   Spicy

Earthy   Herbal

Woodsy

Notes

_____

_____

_____

_____

_____

_____

_____

Effects	Strength				
Peaceful	○	○	○	○	○
Sleepy	○	○	○	○	○
Pain Relief	○	○	○	○	○
Hungry	○	○	○	○	○
Uplifted	○	○	○	○	○
Creative	○	○	○	○	○

Rating ☆ ☆ ☆ ☆ ☆

Strain _____

Grower _____   Date _____

Acquired _____ $ _____

THC % ____	☐ Indica	☐ Flower	Try again?
CBD % ____	☐ Sativa	☐ Edible	☐ Yes
	☐ Hybrid	☐ Concentrate	☐ No

☐ Smoked   ☐ Ate
  ☐ Rolled   ☐ Dabbed
  ☐ Pipe   ☐ Vaped

Symptoms Relieved

_____

_____

_____

_____

_____

Notes

_____

_____

_____

_____

_____

_____

Sweet

Fruity   Floral

Sour   Spicy

Earthy   Herbal

Woodsy

Effects	Strength
Peaceful	◯ ◯ ◯ ◯ ◯
Sleepy	◯ ◯ ◯ ◯ ◯
Pain Relief	◯ ◯ ◯ ◯ ◯
Hungry	◯ ◯ ◯ ◯ ◯
Uplifted	◯ ◯ ◯ ◯ ◯
Creative	◯ ◯ ◯ ◯ ◯

Rating ☆ ☆ ☆ ☆ ☆

Strain

Grower _____ Date _____

Acquired _____ $ _____

THC % ____
CBD % ____

- [ ] Indica
- [ ] Sativa
- [ ] Hybrid

- [ ] Flower
- [ ] Edible
- [ ] Concentrate

Try again?
- [ ] Yes
- [ ] No

- [ ] Smoked
  - [ ] Rolled
  - [ ] Pipe
- [ ] Ate
- [ ] Dabbed
- [ ] Vaped

Symptoms Relieved

_____

_____

_____

_____

_____

Notes

_____

_____

_____

_____

_____

_____

Sweet

Fruity   Floral

Sour   Spicy

Earthy   Herbal

Woodsy

Effects	Strength				
Peaceful	○	○	○	○	○
Sleepy	○	○	○	○	○
Pain Relief	○	○	○	○	○
Hungry	○	○	○	○	○
Uplifted	○	○	○	○	○
Creative	○	○	○	○	○

Rating ☆ ☆ ☆ ☆ ☆

Strain _____

Grower _____ Date _____

Acquired _____ $ _____

THC % ____
CBD % ____

- [ ] Indica
- [ ] Sativa
- [ ] Hybrid

- [ ] Flower
- [ ] Edible
- [ ] Concentrate

Try again?
- [ ] Yes
- [ ] No

- [ ] Smoked
  - [ ] Rolled
  - [ ] Pipe
- [ ] Ate
- [ ] Dabbed
- [ ] Vaped

Symptoms Relieved

_____

_____

_____

_____

_____

Notes

_____

_____

_____

_____

_____

Sweet

Fruity   Floral

Sour   Spicy

Earthy   Herbal

Woodsy

Effects	Strength				
Peaceful	○	○	○	○	○
Sleepy	○	○	○	○	○
Pain Relief	○	○	○	○	○
Hungry	○	○	○	○	○
Uplifted	○	○	○	○	○
Creative	○	○	○	○	○

Rating ☆ ☆ ☆ ☆ ☆

Strain _____

Grower _____ Date _____

Acquired _____ $ _____

THC % ____
CBD % ____

- [ ] Indica
- [ ] Sativa
- [ ] Hybrid

- [ ] Flower
- [ ] Edible
- [ ] Concentrate

Try again?
- [ ] Yes
- [ ] No

- [ ] Smoked
  - [ ] Rolled
  - [ ] Pipe
- [ ] Ate
- [ ] Dabbed
- [ ] Vaped

Symptoms Relieved

_____

_____

_____

_____

_____

Sweet
Fruity   Floral
Sour   Spicy
Earthy   Herbal
Woodsy

Notes

_____

_____

_____

_____

_____

_____

Effects	Strength				
Peaceful	○	○	○	○	○
Sleepy	○	○	○	○	○
Pain Relief	○	○	○	○	○
Hungry	○	○	○	○	○
Uplifted	○	○	○	○	○
Creative	○	○	○	○	○

Rating ☆ ☆ ☆ ☆ ☆

Strain _____

Grower _____   Date _____

Acquired _____ $ _____

THC % ____	☐ Indica	☐ Flower	Try again?
CBD % ____	☐ Sativa	☐ Edible	☐ Yes
	☐ Hybrid	☐ Concentrate	☐ No

☐ Smoked   ☐ Ate
  ☐ Rolled   ☐ Dabbed
  ☐ Pipe   ☐ Vaped

Symptoms Relieved

_____
_____
_____
_____
_____

Sweet

Fruity   Floral

Sour   Spicy

Earthy   Herbal

Woodsy

Notes

_____
_____
_____
_____
_____
_____

Effects	Strength
Peaceful	◯ ◯ ◯ ◯ ◯
Sleepy	◯ ◯ ◯ ◯ ◯
Pain Relief	◯ ◯ ◯ ◯ ◯
Hungry	◯ ◯ ◯ ◯ ◯
Uplifted	◯ ◯ ◯ ◯ ◯
Creative	◯ ◯ ◯ ◯ ◯

Rating ☆ ☆ ☆ ☆ ☆

Strain _____

Grower _____   Date _____

Acquired _____ $ _____

THC % ____	☐ Indica	☐ Flower	Try again?
CBD % ____	☐ Sativa	☐ Edible	☐ Yes
	☐ Hybrid	☐ Concentrate	☐ No

☐ Smoked   ☐ Ate
  ☐ Rolled   ☐ Dabbed
  ☐ Pipe   ☐ Vaped

Symptoms Relieved

_____

_____

_____

_____

_____

Sweet

Fruity   Floral

Sour   Spicy

Earthy   Herbal

Woodsy

Notes

_____

_____

_____

_____

_____

_____

Effects	Strength
Peaceful	○ ○ ○ ○ ○
Sleepy	○ ○ ○ ○ ○
Pain Relief	○ ○ ○ ○ ○
Hungry	○ ○ ○ ○ ○
Uplifted	○ ○ ○ ○ ○
Creative	○ ○ ○ ○ ○

Rating ☆ ☆ ☆ ☆ ☆

Strain _____

Grower _____ Date _____

Acquired _____ $ _____

THC % ____	☐ Indica	☐ Flower	Try again?
CBD % ____	☐ Sativa	☐ Edible	☐ Yes
	☐ Hybrid	☐ Concentrate	☐ No

☐ Smoked	☐ Ate
☐ Rolled	☐ Dabbed
☐ Pipe	☐ Vaped

Symptoms Relieved

_____

_____

_____

_____

_____

Sweet
Fruity   Floral
Sour   Spicy
Earthy   Herbal
Woodsy

Notes

_____

_____

_____

_____

_____

_____

Effects	Strength
Peaceful	○ ○ ○ ○ ○
Sleepy	○ ○ ○ ○ ○
Pain Relief	○ ○ ○ ○ ○
Hungry	○ ○ ○ ○ ○
Uplifted	○ ○ ○ ○ ○
Creative	○ ○ ○ ○ ○

Rating ☆ ☆ ☆ ☆ ☆

Strain _____

Grower _____ Date _____

Acquired _____ $ _____

THC % ____
CBD % ____

- [ ] Indica
- [ ] Sativa
- [ ] Hybrid

- [ ] Flower
- [ ] Edible
- [ ] Concentrate

Try again?
- [ ] Yes
- [ ] No

- [ ] Smoked
  - [ ] Rolled
  - [ ] Pipe
- [ ] Ate
- [ ] Dabbed
- [ ] Vaped

Symptoms Relieved

_____

_____

_____

_____

Notes

_____

_____

_____

_____

_____

_____

Sweet

Fruity

Floral

Sour

Spicy

Earthy

Herbal

Woodsy

Effects	Strength
Peaceful	○ ○ ○ ○ ○
Sleepy	○ ○ ○ ○ ○
Pain Relief	○ ○ ○ ○ ○
Hungry	○ ○ ○ ○ ○
Uplifted	○ ○ ○ ○ ○
Creative	○ ○ ○ ○ ○

Rating ☆ ☆ ☆ ☆ ☆

Strain _____

Grower _____ Date _____

Acquired _____ $ _____

THC % ____
CBD % ____

- [ ] Indica
- [ ] Sativa
- [ ] Hybrid

- [ ] Flower
- [ ] Edible
- [ ] Concentrate

Try again?
- [ ] Yes
- [ ] No

- [ ] Smoked
  - [ ] Rolled
  - [ ] Pipe
- [ ] Ate
- [ ] Dabbed
- [ ] Vaped

Symptoms Relieved

_____

_____

_____

_____

_____

Sweet
Fruity
Floral
Sour
Spicy
Earthy
Herbal
Woodsy

Notes

_____

_____

_____

_____

_____

_____

Effects	Strength				
Peaceful	○	○	○	○	○
Sleepy	○	○	○	○	○
Pain Relief	○	○	○	○	○
Hungry	○	○	○	○	○
Uplifted	○	○	○	○	○
Creative	○	○	○	○	○

Rating ☆ ☆ ☆ ☆ ☆

Strain _____

Grower _____   Date _____

Acquired _____ $ _____

THC % ____   ☐ Indica   ☐ Flower   Try again?
                ☐ Sativa   ☐ Edible   ☐ Yes
CBD % ____   ☐ Hybrid   ☐ Concentrate   ☐ No

☐ Smoked   ☐ Ate
   ☐ Rolled   ☐ Dabbed
   ☐ Pipe   ☐ Vaped

Sweet

Fruity   Floral

Symptoms Relieved

Sour   Spicy

_____

_____

_____   Earthy   Herbal

_____

_____   Woodsy

Effects	Strength				
Peaceful	○	○	○	○	○
## Notes	Sleepy	○	○	○	○	○
Pain Relief	○	○	○	○	○
_____	Hungry	○	○	○	○	○
Uplifted	○	○	○	○	○
_____ | Creative | ○ | ○ | ○ | ○ | ○ |

_____

_____   Rating ☆ ☆ ☆ ☆ ☆

_____

_____

Strain

Grower _____   Date _____

Acquired _____ $ _____

THC % ___
CBD % ___

- [ ] Indica
- [ ] Sativa
- [ ] Hybrid

- [ ] Flower
- [ ] Edible
- [ ] Concentrate

Try again?
- [ ] Yes
- [ ] No

- [ ] Smoked
  - [ ] Rolled
  - [ ] Pipe
- [ ] Ate
- [ ] Dabbed
- [ ] Vaped

Symptoms Relieved

_____

_____

_____

_____

_____

Notes

_____

_____

_____

_____

_____

_____

Sweet

Fruity   Floral

Sour   Spicy

Earthy   Herbal

Woodsy

Effects	Strength				
Peaceful	◯	◯	◯	◯	◯
Sleepy	◯	◯	◯	◯	◯
Pain Relief	◯	◯	◯	◯	◯
Hungry	◯	◯	◯	◯	◯
Uplifted	◯	◯	◯	◯	◯
Creative	◯	◯	◯	◯	◯

Rating ☆ ☆ ☆ ☆ ☆

Strain

Grower _____ Date _____

Acquired _____ $ _____

THC % ____
CBD % ____

☐ Indica
☐ Sativa
☐ Hybrid

☐ Flower
☐ Edible
☐ Concentrate

Try again?
☐ Yes
☐ No

☐ Smoked
  ☐ Rolled
  ☐ Pipe

☐ Ate
☐ Dabbed
☐ Vaped

Symptoms Relieved

_____

_____

_____

_____

_____

Notes

_____

_____

_____

_____

_____

_____

Sweet

Fruity

Floral

Sour

Spicy

Earthy

Herbal

Woodsy

Effects	Strength				
Peaceful	○	○	○	○	○
Sleepy	○	○	○	○	○
Pain Relief	○	○	○	○	○
Hungry	○	○	○	○	○
Uplifted	○	○	○	○	○
Creative	○	○	○	○	○

Rating ☆ ☆ ☆ ☆ ☆

Strain _____

Grower _____   Date _____

Acquired _____ $ _____

| THC % ___ CBD % ___ | ☐ Indica ☐ Sativa ☐ Hybrid | ☐ Flower ☐ Edible ☐ Concentrate | Try again? ☐ Yes ☐ No |

☐ Smoked   ☐ Ate
  ☐ Rolled   ☐ Dabbed
  ☐ Pipe   ☐ Vaped

Symptoms Relieved

_____

_____

_____

_____

_____

Sweet

Fruity   Floral

Sour   Spicy

Earthy   Herbal

Woodsy

Notes

_____

_____

_____

_____

_____

Effects	Strength
Peaceful	○ ○ ○ ○ ○
Sleepy	○ ○ ○ ○ ○
Pain Relief	○ ○ ○ ○ ○
Hungry	○ ○ ○ ○ ○
Uplifted	○ ○ ○ ○ ○
Creative	○ ○ ○ ○ ○

Rating ☆ ☆ ☆ ☆ ☆

Strain _____

Grower _____ Date _____

Acquired _____ $ _____

THC % ____
CBD % ____

- [ ] Indica
- [ ] Sativa
- [ ] Hybrid

- [ ] Flower
- [ ] Edible
- [ ] Concentrate

Try again?
- [ ] Yes
- [ ] No

- [ ] Smoked
  - [ ] Rolled
  - [ ] Pipe
- [ ] Ate
- [ ] Dabbed
- [ ] Vaped

Symptoms Relieved

_____

_____

_____

_____

_____

Sweet

Fruity   Floral

Sour   Spicy

Earthy   Herbal

Woodsy

Notes

_____

_____

_____

_____

_____

_____

Effects	Strength				
Peaceful	○	○	○	○	○
Sleepy	○	○	○	○	○
Pain Relief	○	○	○	○	○
Hungry	○	○	○	○	○
Uplifted	○	○	○	○	○
Creative	○	○	○	○	○

Rating ☆ ☆ ☆ ☆ ☆

Strain _____

Grower _____ Date _____

Acquired _____ $ _____

THC % ____
CBD % ____

- [ ] Indica
- [ ] Sativa
- [ ] Hybrid

- [ ] Flower
- [ ] Edible
- [ ] Concentrate

Try again?
- [ ] Yes
- [ ] No

- [ ] Smoked
  - [ ] Rolled
  - [ ] Pipe
- [ ] Ate
- [ ] Dabbed
- [ ] Vaped

Symptoms Relieved

_____

_____

_____

_____

_____

Sweet

Fruity

Floral

Sour

Spicy

Earthy

Herbal

Woodsy

Notes

_____

_____

_____

_____

_____

_____

Effects	Strength				
Peaceful	○	○	○	○	○
Sleepy	○	○	○	○	○
Pain Relief	○	○	○	○	○
Hungry	○	○	○	○	○
Uplifted	○	○	○	○	○
Creative	○	○	○	○	○

Rating ☆ ☆ ☆ ☆ ☆

Strain _____

Grower _____   Date _____

Acquired _____ $ _____

THC % ____ CBD % ____	☐ Indica ☐ Sativa ☐ Hybrid	☐ Flower ☐ Edible ☐ Concentrate	**Try again?** ☐ Yes ☐ No

☐ Smoked   ☐ Ate
   ☐ Rolled   ☐ Dabbed
   ☐ Pipe   ☐ Vaped

Symptoms Relieved

_____

_____

_____

_____

_____

Sweet

Fruity   Floral

Sour   Spicy

Earthy   Herbal

Woodsy

Notes

_____

_____

_____

_____

_____

_____

Effects	Strength
Peaceful	○ ○ ○ ○ ○
Sleepy	○ ○ ○ ○ ○
Pain Relief	○ ○ ○ ○ ○
Hungry	○ ○ ○ ○ ○
Uplifted	○ ○ ○ ○ ○
Creative	○ ○ ○ ○ ○

Rating ☆ ☆ ☆ ☆ ☆

Strain _____

Grower _____   Date _____

Acquired _____ $ _____

THC % ____
CBD % ____

- [ ] Indica
- [ ] Sativa
- [ ] Hybrid

- [ ] Flower
- [ ] Edible
- [ ] Concentrate

Try again?
- [ ] Yes
- [ ] No

- [ ] Smoked
  - [ ] Rolled
  - [ ] Pipe
- [ ] Ate
- [ ] Dabbed
- [ ] Vaped

Symptoms Relieved

_____

_____

_____

_____

_____

Sweet

Fruity   Floral

Sour   Spicy

Earthy   Herbal

Woodsy

Notes

_____

_____

_____

_____

_____

_____

Effects	Strength				
Peaceful	○	○	○	○	○
Sleepy	○	○	○	○	○
Pain Relief	○	○	○	○	○
Hungry	○	○	○	○	○
Uplifted	○	○	○	○	○
Creative	○	○	○	○	○

Rating ☆ ☆ ☆ ☆ ☆

Strain _____

Grower _____   Date _____

Acquired _____ $ _____

THC % ___	☐ Indica	☐ Flower	Try again?
CBD % ___	☐ Sativa	☐ Edible	☐ Yes
	☐ Hybrid	☐ Concentrate	☐ No

☐ Smoked   ☐ Ate
  ☐ Rolled   ☐ Dabbed
  ☐ Pipe   ☐ Vaped

Symptoms Relieved

_____
_____
_____
_____
_____

Notes

_____
_____
_____
_____
_____
_____

Sweet

Fruity   Floral

Sour   Spicy

Earthy   Herbal

Woodsy

Effects	Strength
Peaceful	○ ○ ○ ○ ○
Sleepy	○ ○ ○ ○ ○
Pain Relief	○ ○ ○ ○ ○
Hungry	○ ○ ○ ○ ○
Uplifted	○ ○ ○ ○ ○
Creative	○ ○ ○ ○ ○

Rating ☆ ☆ ☆ ☆ ☆

Strain _____

Grower _____   Date _____

Acquired _____ $ _____

THC % ___ CBD % ___	☐ Indica ☐ Sativa ☐ Hybrid	☐ Flower ☐ Edible ☐ Concentrate	Try again? ☐ Yes ☐ No

☐ Smoked   ☐ Ate
☐ Rolled   ☐ Dabbed
☐ Pipe   ☐ Vaped

Symptoms Relieved

_____

_____

_____

_____

Sweet

Fruity   Floral

Sour   Spicy

Earthy   Herbal

Woodsy

Notes

_____

_____

_____

_____

_____

Effects	Strength
Peaceful	○ ○ ○ ○ ○
Sleepy	○ ○ ○ ○ ○
Pain Relief	○ ○ ○ ○ ○
Hungry	○ ○ ○ ○ ○
Uplifted	○ ○ ○ ○ ○
Creative	○ ○ ○ ○ ○

Rating ☆ ☆ ☆ ☆ ☆

Strain _____

Grower _____ Date _____

Acquired _____ $ _____

THC % ____
CBD % ____

- [ ] Indica
- [ ] Sativa
- [ ] Hybrid

- [ ] Flower
- [ ] Edible
- [ ] Concentrate

Try again?
- [ ] Yes
- [ ] No

- [ ] Smoked
  - [ ] Rolled
  - [ ] Pipe
- [ ] Ate
- [ ] Dabbed
- [ ] Vaped

Symptoms Relieved

_____
_____
_____
_____
_____

Sweet

Fruity

Floral

Sour

Spicy

Earthy

Herbal

Woodsy

Notes

_____
_____
_____
_____
_____
_____

Effects	Strength				
Peaceful	○	○	○	○	○
Sleepy	○	○	○	○	○
Pain Relief	○	○	○	○	○
Hungry	○	○	○	○	○
Uplifted	○	○	○	○	○
Creative	○	○	○	○	○

Rating ☆ ☆ ☆ ☆ ☆

Strain

Grower _____   Date _____

Acquired _____ $ _____

THC % ____	☐ Indica	☐ Flower	Try again?
CBD % ____	☐ Sativa	☐ Edible	☐ Yes
	☐ Hybrid	☐ Concentrate	☐ No

☐ Smoked   ☐ Ate
  ☐ Rolled   ☐ Dabbed
  ☐ Pipe   ☐ Vaped

Symptoms Relieved

_____

_____

_____

_____

_____

Sweet

Fruity   Floral

Sour   Spicy

Earthy   Herbal

Woodsy

Notes

_____

_____

_____

_____

_____

_____

Effects	Strength				
Peaceful	○	○	○	○	○
Sleepy	○	○	○	○	○
Pain Relief	○	○	○	○	○
Hungry	○	○	○	○	○
Uplifted	○	○	○	○	○
Creative	○	○	○	○	○

Rating ☆ ☆ ☆ ☆ ☆

Strain _____

Grower _____   Date _____

Acquired _____ $ _____

THC % ____
CBD % ____

- [ ] Indica
- [ ] Sativa
- [ ] Hybrid

- [ ] Flower
- [ ] Edible
- [ ] Concentrate

Try again?
- [ ] Yes
- [ ] No

- [ ] Smoked
  - [ ] Rolled
  - [ ] Pipe
- [ ] Ate
- [ ] Dabbed
- [ ] Vaped

Symptoms Relieved

_____

_____

_____

_____

Sweet

Fruity

Floral

Sour

Spicy

Earthy

Herbal

Woodsy

Notes

_____

_____

_____

_____

_____

_____

Effects	Strength				
Peaceful	○	○	○	○	○
Sleepy	○	○	○	○	○
Pain Relief	○	○	○	○	○
Hungry	○	○	○	○	○
Uplifted	○	○	○	○	○
Creative	○	○	○	○	○

Rating ☆ ☆ ☆ ☆ ☆

Strain

Grower _____   Date _____

Acquired _____ $ _____

THC % ___	☐ Indica	☐ Flower	Try again?
CBD % ___	☐ Sativa	☐ Edible	☐ Yes
	☐ Hybrid	☐ Concentrate	☐ No

☐ Smoked   ☐ Ate
  ☐ Rolled   ☐ Dabbed
  ☐ Pipe   ☐ Vaped

Symptoms Relieved

_____

_____

_____

_____

_____

Sweet
Fruity
Floral
Sour
Spicy
Earthy
Herbal
Woodsy

Effects	Strength
Peaceful	○ ○ ○ ○ ○
Sleepy	○ ○ ○ ○ ○
Pain Relief	○ ○ ○ ○ ○
Hungry	○ ○ ○ ○ ○
Uplifted	○ ○ ○ ○ ○
Creative	○ ○ ○ ○ ○

Notes

_____

_____

_____

_____

_____

Rating ☆ ☆ ☆ ☆ ☆

Strain _____

Grower _____ Date _____

Acquired _____ $ _____

THC % ___ CBD % ___	☐ Indica ☐ Sativa ☐ Hybrid

☐ Flower   ☐ Edible   ☐ Concentrate

Try again?
☐ Yes
☐ No

☐ Smoked   ☐ Ate
   ☐ Rolled   ☐ Dabbed
   ☐ Pipe   ☐ Vaped

Symptoms Relieved

_____

_____

_____

_____

Sweet

Fruity

Floral

Sour

Spicy

Earthy

Herbal

Woodsy

Notes

_____

_____

_____

_____

_____

_____

Effects	Strength
Peaceful	○ ○ ○ ○ ○
Sleepy	○ ○ ○ ○ ○
Pain Relief	○ ○ ○ ○ ○
Hungry	○ ○ ○ ○ ○
Uplifted	○ ○ ○ ○ ○
Creative	○ ○ ○ ○ ○

Rating ☆ ☆ ☆ ☆ ☆

Strain

Grower _____   Date _____

Acquired _____ $ _____

THC % _____
CBD % _____

- [ ] Indica
- [ ] Sativa
- [ ] Hybrid

- [ ] Flower
- [ ] Edible
- [ ] Concentrate

Try again?
- [ ] Yes
- [ ] No

- [ ] Smoked
  - [ ] Rolled
  - [ ] Pipe
- [ ] Ate
- [ ] Dabbed
- [ ] Vaped

Symptoms Relieved

_____

_____

_____

_____

_____

Sweet
Fruity   Floral
Sour   Spicy
Earthy   Herbal
Woodsy

Notes

_____

_____

_____

_____

_____

_____

Effects	Strength				
Peaceful	○	○	○	○	○
Sleepy	○	○	○	○	○
Pain Relief	○	○	○	○	○
Hungry	○	○	○	○	○
Uplifted	○	○	○	○	○
Creative	○	○	○	○	○

Rating ☆ ☆ ☆ ☆ ☆

Strain _____

Grower _____   Date _____

Acquired _____ $ _____

THC % ___	☐ Indica	☐ Flower	Try again?
CBD % ___	☐ Sativa	☐ Edible	☐ Yes
	☐ Hybrid	☐ Concentrate	☐ No

☐ Smoked   ☐ Ate
  ☐ Rolled   ☐ Dabbed
  ☐ Pipe   ☐ Vaped

Symptoms Relieved

_____

_____

_____

_____

_____

Notes

_____

_____

_____

_____

_____

_____

Sweet

Fruity   Floral

Sour   Spicy

Earthy   Herbal

Woodsy

Effects	Strength
Peaceful	○ ○ ○ ○ ○
Sleepy	○ ○ ○ ○ ○
Pain Relief	○ ○ ○ ○ ○
Hungry	○ ○ ○ ○ ○
Uplifted	○ ○ ○ ○ ○
Creative	○ ○ ○ ○ ○

Rating ☆ ☆ ☆ ☆ ☆

Strain _____

Grower _____   Date _____

Acquired _____ $ _____

THC % ___	☐ Indica	☐ Flower	Try again?
CBD % ___	☐ Sativa	☐ Edible	☐ Yes
	☐ Hybrid	☐ Concentrate	☐ No

☐ Smoked   ☐ Ate
  ☐ Rolled   ☐ Dabbed
  ☐ Pipe   ☐ Vaped

Sweet
Fruity
Floral
Sour
Spicy
Earthy
Herbal
Woodsy

Symptoms Relieved

_____

_____

_____

_____

_____

Notes

_____

_____

_____

_____

_____

_____

Effects	Strength
Peaceful	○ ○ ○ ○ ○
Sleepy	○ ○ ○ ○ ○
Pain Relief	○ ○ ○ ○ ○
Hungry	○ ○ ○ ○ ○
Uplifted	○ ○ ○ ○ ○
Creative	○ ○ ○ ○ ○

Rating ☆ ☆ ☆ ☆ ☆

Strain _____

Grower _____   Date _____

Acquired _____ $ _____

THC % ____ CBD % ____	☐ Indica ☐ Sativa ☐ Hybrid	☐ Flower ☐ Edible ☐ Concentrate	Try again? ☐ Yes ☐ No

☐ Smoked   ☐ Ate
  ☐ Rolled   ☐ Dabbed
  ☐ Pipe   ☐ Vaped

Symptoms Relieved

_____

_____

_____

_____

_____

Sweet

Fruity   Floral

Sour   Spicy

Earthy   Herbal

Woodsy

Notes

_____

_____

_____

_____

_____

_____

Effects	Strength
Peaceful	○ ○ ○ ○ ○
Sleepy	○ ○ ○ ○ ○
Pain Relief	○ ○ ○ ○ ○
Hungry	○ ○ ○ ○ ○
Uplifted	○ ○ ○ ○ ○
Creative	○ ○ ○ ○ ○

Rating ☆ ☆ ☆ ☆ ☆

Strain

Grower _____ Date _____

Acquired _____ $ _____

THC % ____
CBD % ____

- [ ] Indica
- [ ] Sativa
- [ ] Hybrid

- [ ] Flower
- [ ] Edible
- [ ] Concentrate

Try again?
- [ ] Yes
- [ ] No

- [ ] Smoked
  - [ ] Rolled
  - [ ] Pipe
- [ ] Ate
- [ ] Dabbed
- [ ] Vaped

Symptoms Relieved

_____

_____

_____

_____

Sweet

Fruity

Floral

Sour

Spicy

Earthy

Herbal

Woodsy

Notes

_____

_____

_____

_____

_____

Effects	Strength				
Peaceful	○	○	○	○	○
Sleepy	○	○	○	○	○
Pain Relief	○	○	○	○	○
Hungry	○	○	○	○	○
Uplifted	○	○	○	○	○
Creative	○	○	○	○	○

Rating ☆ ☆ ☆ ☆ ☆

Strain _____

Grower _____ Date _____

Acquired _____ $ _____

THC % ____	☐ Indica	☐ Flower	Try again?
CBD % ____	☐ Sativa	☐ Edible	☐ Yes
	☐ Hybrid	☐ Concentrate	☐ No

☐ Smoked   ☐ Ate
  ☐ Rolled   ☐ Dabbed
  ☐ Pipe   ☐ Vaped

Symptoms Relieved

_____

_____

_____

_____

_____

Notes

_____

_____

_____

_____

_____

_____

Sweet

Fruity   Floral

Sour   Spicy

Earthy   Herbal

Woodsy

Effects	Strength
Peaceful	○ ○ ○ ○ ○
Sleepy	○ ○ ○ ○ ○
Pain Relief	○ ○ ○ ○ ○
Hungry	○ ○ ○ ○ ○
Uplifted	○ ○ ○ ○ ○
Creative	○ ○ ○ ○ ○

Rating ☆ ☆ ☆ ☆ ☆

Strain

Grower _____ Date _____

Acquired _____ $ _____

THC % ____
CBD % ____

- [ ] Indica
- [ ] Sativa
- [ ] Hybrid

- [ ] Flower
- [ ] Edible
- [ ] Concentrate

Try again?
- [ ] Yes
- [ ] No

- [ ] Smoked
  - [ ] Rolled
  - [ ] Pipe
- [ ] Ate
- [ ] Dabbed
- [ ] Vaped

Symptoms Relieved

_____

_____

_____

_____

_____

Sweet

Fruity   Floral

Sour   Spicy

Earthy   Herbal

Woodsy

Notes

_____

_____

_____

_____

_____

Effects	Strength				
Peaceful	○	○	○	○	○
Sleepy	○	○	○	○	○
Pain Relief	○	○	○	○	○
Hungry	○	○	○	○	○
Uplifted	○	○	○	○	○
Creative	○	○	○	○	○

Rating ☆ ☆ ☆ ☆ ☆

Strain _____

Grower _____ Date _____

Acquired _____ $ _____

THC % ____	☐ Indica	☐ Flower	Try again?
CBD % ____	☐ Sativa	☐ Edible	☐ Yes
	☐ Hybrid	☐ Concentrate	☐ No

☐ Smoked   ☐ Ate
  ☐ Rolled   ☐ Dabbed
  ☐ Pipe   ☐ Vaped

Symptoms Relieved

_____

_____

_____

_____

Notes

_____

_____

_____

_____

_____

_____

Sweet

Fruity   Floral

Sour   Spicy

Earthy   Herbal

Woodsy

Effects	Strength
Peaceful	○ ○ ○ ○ ○
Sleepy	○ ○ ○ ○ ○
Pain Relief	○ ○ ○ ○ ○
Hungry	○ ○ ○ ○ ○
Uplifted	○ ○ ○ ○ ○
Creative	○ ○ ○ ○ ○

Rating ☆ ☆ ☆ ☆ ☆

Strain _____

Grower _____ Date _____

Acquired _____ $ _____

THC % ___	☐ Indica	☐ Flower	Try again?
CBD % ___	☐ Sativa	☐ Edible	☐ Yes
	☐ Hybrid	☐ Concentrate	☐ No

☐ Smoked   ☐ Ate
  ☐ Rolled   ☐ Dabbed
  ☐ Pipe   ☐ Vaped

Symptoms Relieved

_____

_____

_____

_____

_____

Notes

_____

_____

_____

_____

_____

_____

Sweet

Fruity   Floral

Sour   Spicy

Earthy   Herbal

Woodsy

Effects	Strength
Peaceful	○ ○ ○ ○ ○
Sleepy	○ ○ ○ ○ ○
Pain Relief	○ ○ ○ ○ ○
Hungry	○ ○ ○ ○ ○
Uplifted	○ ○ ○ ○ ○
Creative	○ ○ ○ ○ ○

Rating ☆ ☆ ☆ ☆ ☆

Strain _____

Grower _____ Date _____

Acquired _____ $ _____

THC % ____	☐ Indica	☐ Flower	Try again?
CBD % ____	☐ Sativa	☐ Edible	☐ Yes
	☐ Hybrid	☐ Concentrate	☐ No

☐ Smoked   ☐ Ate
  ☐ Rolled   ☐ Dabbed
  ☐ Pipe   ☐ Vaped

Symptoms Relieved

_____

_____

_____

_____

_____

Notes

_____

_____

_____

_____

_____

_____

Sweet

Fruity   Floral

Sour   Spicy

Earthy   Herbal

Woodsy

Effects	Strength
Peaceful	○ ○ ○ ○ ○
Sleepy	○ ○ ○ ○ ○
Pain Relief	○ ○ ○ ○ ○
Hungry	○ ○ ○ ○ ○
Uplifted	○ ○ ○ ○ ○
Creative	○ ○ ○ ○ ○

Rating ☆ ☆ ☆ ☆ ☆

Strain _____

Grower _____   Date _____

Acquired _____ $ _____

THC % ___	☐ Indica	☐ Flower	Try again?
CBD % ___	☐ Sativa	☐ Edible	☐ Yes
	☐ Hybrid	☐ Concentrate	☐ No

☐ Smoked   ☐ Ate
　☐ Rolled   ☐ Dabbed
　☐ Pipe   ☐ Vaped

Symptoms Relieved

_____

_____

_____

_____

Sweet

Fruity   Floral

Sour   Spicy

Earthy   Herbal

Woodsy

Notes

_____

_____

_____

_____

_____

_____

Effects	Strength
Peaceful	○ ○ ○ ○ ○
Sleepy	○ ○ ○ ○ ○
Pain Relief	○ ○ ○ ○ ○
Hungry	○ ○ ○ ○ ○
Uplifted	○ ○ ○ ○ ○
Creative	○ ○ ○ ○ ○

Rating ☆ ☆ ☆ ☆ ☆

Strain _____

Grower _____   Date _____

Acquired _____ $ _____

THC % ___	☐ Indica	☐ Flower	Try again?
CBD % ___	☐ Sativa	☐ Edible	☐ Yes
	☐ Hybrid	☐ Concentrate	☐ No

☐ Smoked   ☐ Ate
  ☐ Rolled   ☐ Dabbed
  ☐ Pipe   ☐ Vaped

Sweet

Fruity   Floral

Sour   Spicy

Earthy   Herbal

Woodsy

Symptoms Relieved

_____

_____

_____

_____

_____

Effects	Strength
Peaceful	○ ○ ○ ○ ○
Sleepy	○ ○ ○ ○ ○
Pain Relief	○ ○ ○ ○ ○
Hungry	○ ○ ○ ○ ○
Uplifted	○ ○ ○ ○ ○
Creative	○ ○ ○ ○ ○

Notes

_____

_____

_____

_____

_____

_____

Rating ☆ ☆ ☆ ☆ ☆

Strain _____

Grower _____   Date _____

Acquired _____ $ _____

THC % ___	☐ Indica	☐ Flower	Try again?
CBD % ___	☐ Sativa	☐ Edible	☐ Yes
	☐ Hybrid	☐ Concentrate	☐ No

☐ Smoked   ☐ Ate
  ☐ Rolled   ☐ Dabbed
  ☐ Pipe   ☐ Vaped

Symptoms Relieved

_____

_____

_____

_____

Sweet

Fruity   Floral

Sour   Spicy

Earthy   Herbal

Woodsy

Notes

_____

_____

_____

_____

_____

Effects	Strength				
Peaceful	○	○	○	○	○
Sleepy	○	○	○	○	○
Pain Relief	○	○	○	○	○
Hungry	○	○	○	○	○
Uplifted	○	○	○	○	○
Creative	○	○	○	○	○

Rating ☆ ☆ ☆ ☆ ☆

Strain _____

Grower _____ Date _____

Acquired _____ $ _____

THC % ____	☐ Indica	☐ Flower	Try again?
CBD % ____	☐ Sativa	☐ Edible	☐ Yes
	☐ Hybrid	☐ Concentrate	☐ No

☐ Smoked   ☐ Ate
  ☐ Rolled   ☐ Dabbed
  ☐ Pipe   ☐ Vaped

Symptoms Relieved

_____

_____

_____

_____

Notes

_____

_____

_____

_____

_____

Sweet

Fruity   Floral

Sour   Spicy

Earthy   Herbal

Woodsy

Effects	Strength
Peaceful	○ ○ ○ ○ ○
Sleepy	○ ○ ○ ○ ○
Pain Relief	○ ○ ○ ○ ○
Hungry	○ ○ ○ ○ ○
Uplifted	○ ○ ○ ○ ○
Creative	○ ○ ○ ○ ○

Rating ☆ ☆ ☆ ☆ ☆

Strain _____

Grower _____   Date _____

Acquired _____ $ _____

THC % ____	☐ Indica	☐ Flower	Try again?
CBD % ____	☐ Sativa	☐ Edible	☐ Yes
	☐ Hybrid	☐ Concentrate	☐ No

☐ Smoked   ☐ Ate
  ☐ Rolled   ☐ Dabbed
  ☐ Pipe   ☐ Vaped

Symptoms Relieved

_____

_____

_____

_____

_____

Notes

_____

_____

_____

_____

_____

_____

Sweet
Fruity
Floral
Sour
Spicy
Earthy
Herbal
Woodsy

Effects	Strength				
Peaceful	○	○	○	○	○
Sleepy	○	○	○	○	○
Pain Relief	○	○	○	○	○
Hungry	○	○	○	○	○
Uplifted	○	○	○	○	○
Creative	○	○	○	○	○

Rating ☆ ☆ ☆ ☆ ☆

Strain _____

Grower _____   Date _____

Acquired _____ $ _____

THC % ____ CBD % ____	☐ Indica ☐ Sativa ☐ Hybrid	☐ Flower ☐ Edible ☐ Concentrate	Try again? ☐ Yes ☐ No

☐ Smoked ☐ Ate
   ☐ Rolled ☐ Dabbed
   ☐ Pipe ☐ Vaped

Symptoms Relieved

_____

_____

_____

_____

_____

Notes

_____

_____

_____

_____

_____

_____

Sweet
Fruity — Floral
Sour — Spicy
Earthy — Herbal
Woodsy

Effects	Strength
Peaceful	○ ○ ○ ○ ○
Sleepy	○ ○ ○ ○ ○
Pain Relief	○ ○ ○ ○ ○
Hungry	○ ○ ○ ○ ○
Uplifted	○ ○ ○ ○ ○
Creative	○ ○ ○ ○ ○

Rating ☆ ☆ ☆ ☆ ☆

Strain _____

Grower _____ Date _____

Acquired _____ $ _____

THC % ____

CBD % ____

- [ ] Indica
- [ ] Sativa
- [ ] Hybrid

- [ ] Flower
- [ ] Edible
- [ ] Concentrate

Try again?
- [ ] Yes
- [ ] No

- [ ] Smoked
  - [ ] Rolled
  - [ ] Pipe
- [ ] Ate
- [ ] Dabbed
- [ ] Vaped

Symptoms Relieved

_____

_____

_____

_____

_____

Sweet

Fruity   Floral

Sour   Spicy

Earthy   Herbal

Woodsy

Notes

_____

_____

_____

_____

_____

_____

Effects	Strength				
Peaceful	○	○	○	○	○
Sleepy	○	○	○	○	○
Pain Relief	○	○	○	○	○
Hungry	○	○	○	○	○
Uplifted	○	○	○	○	○
Creative	○	○	○	○	○

Rating ☆ ☆ ☆ ☆ ☆

Strain _____

Grower _____ Date _____

Acquired _____ $ _____

THC % ____
CBD % ____

- [ ] Indica
- [ ] Sativa
- [ ] Hybrid

- [ ] Flower
- [ ] Edible
- [ ] Concentrate

Try again?
- [ ] Yes
- [ ] No

- [ ] Smoked
  - [ ] Rolled
  - [ ] Pipe
- [ ] Ate
- [ ] Dabbed
- [ ] Vaped

Sweet

Fruity   Floral

Sour   Spicy

Symptoms Relieved

Earthy   Herbal

_____
_____   Woodsy
_____
_____
_____

Effects	Strength				
Peaceful	◯	◯	◯	◯	◯

Notes

Sleepy	◯	◯	◯	◯	◯
Pain Relief	◯	◯	◯	◯	◯
Hungry	◯	◯	◯	◯	◯
Uplifted	◯	◯	◯	◯	◯
Creative	◯	◯	◯	◯	◯

_____
_____
_____
_____   **Rating** ☆ ☆ ☆ ☆ ☆
_____
_____

Strain _____

Grower _____   Date _____

Acquired _____ $ _____

THC % ____	☐ Indica	☐ Flower	Try again?
CBD % ____	☐ Sativa	☐ Edible	☐ Yes
	☐ Hybrid	☐ Concentrate	☐ No

☐ Smoked   ☐ Ate
  ☐ Rolled   ☐ Dabbed
  ☐ Pipe   ☐ Vaped

Symptoms Relieved

_____

_____

_____

_____

_____

Sweet

Fruity   Floral

Sour   Spicy

Earthy   Herbal

Woodsy

Notes

_____

_____

_____

_____

_____

Effects	Strength
Peaceful	○ ○ ○ ○ ○
Sleepy	○ ○ ○ ○ ○
Pain Relief	○ ○ ○ ○ ○
Hungry	○ ○ ○ ○ ○
Uplifted	○ ○ ○ ○ ○
Creative	○ ○ ○ ○ ○

Rating ☆ ☆ ☆ ☆ ☆

Strain _____

Grower _____ Date _____

Acquired _____ $ _____

THC % ____
CBD % ____

- [ ] Indica
- [ ] Sativa
- [ ] Hybrid

- [ ] Flower
- [ ] Edible
- [ ] Concentrate

Try again?
- [ ] Yes
- [ ] No

- [ ] Smoked
  - [ ] Rolled
  - [ ] Pipe
- [ ] Ate
- [ ] Dabbed
- [ ] Vaped

Symptoms Relieved

_____

_____

_____

_____

_____

Sweet

Fruity   Floral

Sour   Spicy

Earthy   Herbal

Woodsy

Notes

_____

_____

_____

_____

_____

_____

Effects	Strength
Peaceful	○ ○ ○ ○ ○
Sleepy	○ ○ ○ ○ ○
Pain Relief	○ ○ ○ ○ ○
Hungry	○ ○ ○ ○ ○
Uplifted	○ ○ ○ ○ ○
Creative	○ ○ ○ ○ ○

Rating ☆ ☆ ☆ ☆ ☆

Strain _____

Grower _____   Date _____

Acquired _____ $ _____

THC % ____	☐ Indica	☐ Flower	Try again?
CBD % ____	☐ Sativa	☐ Edible	☐ Yes
	☐ Hybrid	☐ Concentrate	☐ No

☐ Smoked   ☐ Ate
　☐ Rolled   ☐ Dabbed
　☐ Pipe   ☐ Vaped

Symptoms Relieved

_____

_____

_____

_____

_____

Sweet

Fruity   Floral

Sour   Spicy

Earthy   Herbal

Woodsy

Notes

_____

_____

_____

_____

_____

_____

Effects	Strength				
Peaceful	◯	◯	◯	◯	◯
Sleepy	◯	◯	◯	◯	◯
Pain Relief	◯	◯	◯	◯	◯
Hungry	◯	◯	◯	◯	◯
Uplifted	◯	◯	◯	◯	◯
Creative	◯	◯	◯	◯	◯

Rating ☆ ☆ ☆ ☆ ☆

Strain _____

Grower _____   Date _____

Acquired _____ $ _____

THC % ___ CBD % ___	☐ Indica ☐ Sativa ☐ Hybrid	☐ Flower ☐ Edible ☐ Concentrate	Try again? ☐ Yes ☐ No

☐ Smoked   ☐ Ate
   ☐ Rolled   ☐ Dabbed
   ☐ Pipe   ☐ Vaped

Symptoms Relieved

_____

_____

_____

_____

Notes

_____

_____

_____

_____

_____

_____

Sweet

Fruity   Floral

Sour   Spicy

Earthy   Herbal

Woodsy

Effects	Strength				
Peaceful	○	○	○	○	○
Sleepy	○	○	○	○	○
Pain Relief	○	○	○	○	○
Hungry	○	○	○	○	○
Uplifted	○	○	○	○	○
Creative	○	○	○	○	○

Rating ☆ ☆ ☆ ☆ ☆

Strain

Grower _____ Date _____

Acquired _____ $ _____

THC % _____
CBD % _____

- [ ] Indica
- [ ] Sativa
- [ ] Hybrid

- [ ] Flower
- [ ] Edible
- [ ] Concentrate

Try again?
- [ ] Yes
- [ ] No

- [ ] Smoked
  - [ ] Rolled
  - [ ] Pipe
- [ ] Ate
- [ ] Dabbed
- [ ] Vaped

Symptoms Relieved

_____

_____

_____

_____

_____

Sweet
Fruity
Floral
Sour
Spicy
Earthy
Herbal
Woodsy

Notes

_____

_____

_____

_____

_____

Effects	Strength				
Peaceful	○	○	○	○	○
Sleepy	○	○	○	○	○
Pain Relief	○	○	○	○	○
Hungry	○	○	○	○	○
Uplifted	○	○	○	○	○
Creative	○	○	○	○	○

Rating ☆ ☆ ☆ ☆ ☆

Strain _____

Grower _____   Date _____

Acquired _____ $ _____

THC % ___	☐ Indica	☐ Flower	Try again?
CBD % ___	☐ Sativa	☐ Edible	☐ Yes
	☐ Hybrid	☐ Concentrate	☐ No

☐ Smoked   ☐ Ate
  ☐ Rolled   ☐ Dabbed
  ☐ Pipe   ☐ Vaped

Symptoms Relieved

_____

_____

_____

_____

_____

Sweet

Fruity   Floral

Sour   Spicy

Earthy   Herbal

Woodsy

Notes

_____

_____

_____

_____

_____

_____

_____

Effects	Strength				
Peaceful	◯	◯	◯	◯	◯
Sleepy	◯	◯	◯	◯	◯
Pain Relief	◯	◯	◯	◯	◯
Hungry	◯	◯	◯	◯	◯
Uplifted	◯	◯	◯	◯	◯
Creative	◯	◯	◯	◯	◯

Rating ☆ ☆ ☆ ☆ ☆

Strain _____

Grower _____ Date _____

Acquired _____ $ _____

THC % ___	☐ Indica	☐ Flower	Try again?
CBD % ___	☐ Sativa	☐ Edible	☐ Yes
	☐ Hybrid	☐ Concentrate	☐ No

☐ Smoked   ☐ Ate
  ☐ Rolled   ☐ Dabbed
  ☐ Pipe   ☐ Vaped

Symptoms Relieved

_____

_____

_____

_____

_____

Notes

_____

_____

_____

_____

_____

_____

Sweet

Fruity

Floral

Sour

Spicy

Earthy

Herbal

Woodsy

Effects	Strength				
Peaceful	○	○	○	○	○
Sleepy	○	○	○	○	○
Pain Relief	○	○	○	○	○
Hungry	○	○	○	○	○
Uplifted	○	○	○	○	○
Creative	○	○	○	○	○

Rating ☆ ☆ ☆ ☆ ☆

Strain _____

Grower _____ Date _____

Acquired _____ $ _____

THC % ____	☐ Indica	☐ Flower	Try again?
CBD % ____	☐ Sativa	☐ Edible	☐ Yes
	☐ Hybrid	☐ Concentrate	☐ No

☐ Smoked ☐ Ate
  ☐ Rolled ☐ Dabbed
  ☐ Pipe ☐ Vaped

Symptoms Relieved

_____

_____

_____

_____

Notes

_____

_____

_____

_____

_____

Sweet

Fruity   Floral

Sour   Spicy

Earthy   Herbal

Woodsy

Effects	Strength				
Peaceful	○	○	○	○	○
Sleepy	○	○	○	○	○
Pain Relief	○	○	○	○	○
Hungry	○	○	○	○	○
Uplifted	○	○	○	○	○
Creative	○	○	○	○	○

Rating ☆ ☆ ☆ ☆ ☆

Strain

Grower _____ Date _____

Acquired _____ $ _____

THC % ___	☐ Indica	☐ Flower	Try again?
CBD % ___	☐ Sativa	☐ Edible	☐ Yes
	☐ Hybrid	☐ Concentrate	☐ No

☐ Smoked ☐ Ate
 ☐ Rolled ☐ Dabbed
 ☐ Pipe ☐ Vaped

Symptoms Relieved

_____

_____

_____

_____

_____

Sweet

Fruity   Floral

Sour   Spicy

Earthy   Herbal

Woodsy

Notes

_____

_____

_____

_____

_____

_____

Effects	Strength
Peaceful	○ ○ ○ ○ ○
Sleepy	○ ○ ○ ○ ○
Pain Relief	○ ○ ○ ○ ○
Hungry	○ ○ ○ ○ ○
Uplifted	○ ○ ○ ○ ○
Creative	○ ○ ○ ○ ○

Rating ☆ ☆ ☆ ☆ ☆

Strain _____

Grower _____ Date _____

Acquired _____ $ _____

THC % ____
CBD % ____

- [ ] Indica
- [ ] Sativa
- [ ] Hybrid

- [ ] Flower
- [ ] Edible
- [ ] Concentrate

Try again?
- [ ] Yes
- [ ] No

- [ ] Smoked
  - [ ] Rolled
  - [ ] Pipe
- [ ] Ate
- [ ] Dabbed
- [ ] Vaped

Symptoms Relieved

_____

_____

_____

_____

_____

Sweet

Fruity   Floral

Sour   Spicy

Earthy   Herbal

Woodsy

Notes

_____

_____

_____

_____

_____

_____

Effects	Strength				
Peaceful	○	○	○	○	○
Sleepy	○	○	○	○	○
Pain Relief	○	○	○	○	○
Hungry	○	○	○	○	○
Uplifted	○	○	○	○	○
Creative	○	○	○	○	○

Rating ☆ ☆ ☆ ☆ ☆

Made in the USA
Monee, IL
11 December 2019